"*Second Story Woman* will resonate with anyone who wants to leave behind their worn out image of who they are and create a new vision for the next phase of their lives. Calladine's voice is authentic, honest and inspiring. Her story is especially empowering for readers challenged with managing their diabetes."

> —Marsha McGregor, essayist and workshop
> facilitator, International Women's Writing Guild

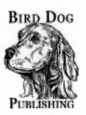

BIRD DOG

PUBLISHING

Second Story Woman

A Memoir of Second Chances

Carole Calladine

For Joyce –
Best Wishes –
Carole Calladine

Bird Dog Publishing
Huron, Ohio

Bird Dog Publishing
PO Box 425/ Huron, OH 44839
http://members.aol.com/Lsmithdog/bottomdog

A division of
Bottom Dog Press
Which is supported in part by
The Ohio Arts Council

All Photographs by Carole Calladine
Author photos by Judy Collins

Acknowledgments

This book is written for all...who want a second chance.

Like all good works of non-fiction, this story is true. But as a therapist, I know it is my truth and others may have a different recollection of the events contained in this book. (They are welcome to write their truths and I will applaud and learn from them when they do so.) However, to protect the confidentiality of the book's "scoundrels," I have changed the names and even the sex of some characters met within these pages, but not their actions. I haven't changed any family or close friends' names and hope they will forgive me for any liberties I have taken in sharing these memories.

My intent is to not embarrass anyone, unless it is myself. I share this journey with hopes of helping others.The social work educator lives on in me. But I must confess that I do have a selfish motive in crafting this book. I want to remember this important decade of my life and dip back into it whenever I land in future "tight" places.

I thank all who supported me during the ten-year journey of living and writing this book. You are too numerous to list, but know in your heart that I couldn't have completed this project without your help and best wishes.

That said, I would like to acknowledge those who were at the finish line holding my hand.

Deanna Adams, a writing partner and member of the M.C. Essayists (Miriam Carey was our teacher) that meets monthly.

Jackie Green, a line editor and friend who is a member of the Saturday Morning Writing group that meets weekly at 7:00 a.m.

Marsha McGregor of the International Women Writers Guild (IWWG) who edited the first section in its infancy and is a member of the Kent IWWG writing group that meets monthly.

Kathleen Forrest, an editor found at the Firelands Writing Center that meets monthly. As associate editor for Bird Dog Publishing, Kathleen graciously accepted the task of reading the final version for clarity and meaning.

Geri Bryan, a best friend and traveling partner to all the above groups. She and my other friends in our Artist Way Cluster group helped me to believe in myself and cheered me on.

Larry Smith and Bird Dog Publishing for accepting and editing this book into a readable memoir. Without his push this book would still be in a three-ring binder.

Michael and Brendan Calladine—fine sons who believe in me unconditionally.

Andrew, my husband of forty years who has always been there, applauded me, and made me feel cherished.

Contents

"The Iliad is only great because all life is a battle, The Odyssey because all life is a journey, the Book of Job because all life is a riddle."
—G. K. Chesterton

Prologue: Second Opinion

"You are out of control," said my internist waving her hands in my face.

I hadn't been good, disciplined, or compliant. I no longer walked after work. If available, I had a donut at my morning coffee break. (I made sure they were available by stopping at Elmwood Bakery on the way to work with the excuse, "They're for the staff.") And the custard stand across from my office building was open for the season. Hot fudge sundae treats called to me when I worked late, which was most evenings.

"You were a star pupil, Carole. Of the sixteen million Americans who have type 2 diabetes, I thought you were one of the lucky ones who was going to beat this disease." She heaped on the guilt. "What happened since your last check-up?"

"Well," I hedged, "I did go on a vacation to Vegas." I jested, "Guess I tripped up after my trip."

She didn't laugh.

"Get it? Tripped up after my trip."

"Right. And the dog ate your homework, too," she gave it right back to me. "What could possibly have happened in Vegas that you've regained nine pounds? And made your A1c a 9 instead of an acceptable 6.5." (The A1c count is a three-month measurement of the amount of glucose that attaches itself to the protein that transports oxygen around the body.) She threw her hands up in the air again. "Unbelievable! You're destroying your body."

Not wanting more excuses, she referred me to Dr. Carey, an endocrinologist, and debated whether or not to put me on insulin. Visions of needles danced in my head. *Ugh!*

Legs dangling over the edge of the black leather gurney, I sat sweating in an XXL cotton gown that thankfully covered all of me. Dr. Carey's exam room had brown plaid carpet and the only decorations were diplomas in utility frames. A sink, tray table, and a straight-back chair completed the "functional only" furnishings. This office was definitely not the sunny country décor of my internist's suite. Even the wall clock had already been changed for the weekend's Daylight Savings Time. *They didn't mess around here.*

Daylight Savings Time. D.S.T. Word play relieves my anxiety so I started fooling around. *Let's see. D.S.T. could stand for Diabetes Saving Time. Dazzling Showgirl Time. Delicious Sundae Treats. Dreams Spell Trouble. Dead Serious Time. Deadly Serious Tasks. Detention Starts Today. Disaster Strikes old-Timer. Deadbeat Seeks Trial. Or, how about Deadly Sweet Tooth?* My anxiety soared. Switching tactics, I took a deep breath, counted to ten, and exhaled. I took another and counted to ten. *Exhale. I choose Dazzling Showgirl Time. Inhale. Exhale. Dazzling Showgirl Time.*

Dr. Carey entered and sat in the straight-back chair. *Wouldn't you know it? She was petite. But then, if she'd been heavy, I wouldn't have been happy either challenging her ability to treat an overweight diabetic.*

Her husky voice filled the room as she asked questions, writing in long hand on narrow-ruled, notebook paper. I answered.

"No. No diabetic history in the family. I'm the first."

"Yes, my mom had an overactive thyroid removed and she died two years ago of Lou Gehrig's disease."

"Yes, my dad has high blood pressure, macular degeneration, and is still living."

Dead Serious Time.

"Both my maternal grandparents died of heart attacks."

"My grandfather wasn't overweight, but yes, my maternal grandmother was. No, she'd never been diagnosed with diabetes.

"I never knew my paternal grandparents. But my dad's mom died young of pneumonia. And my dad's father drank himself into old age, living into his nineties."

Disaster Strikes old-Timer.

Finished with my family history, she began her physical examination.

"Take a deep breath and hold it."

I held it. *Diabetes Saving Time.*

She placed cool hands on my hot menopausal skin, kneading my internal body organs. She put buzzing mechanical devices against the bottoms of my feet and asked me if I could feel them.

"Yes...Yes." *Why wouldn't I be able to feel them?* Regardless of why, I thanked God that I could. "Yes."

Deadbeat Seeks Trial.

"You're carrying extra weight in your abdomen. It needs to come off." She turned to leave, "Dress, and then join me in the office. We'll talk."

Detention Starts Today.

In her office, behind a metal desk with her notes, lab reports, and the internist's consult request, Dr. Carey reviewed my medical condition. I mainly listened because I was on my best behavior, still nervous around this straight talking doctor.

Finally I ventured forth with a question. "What weight loss program do you recommend?"

"I recommend keeping a food diary and recording everything you put in your mouth, even a piece of gum," she left no room for argument. "You'll know soon enough what to eat. And, if you need a weekly weigh-in to keep you honest, my nurse will weigh you every week for free."

"No. No, that won't be necessary."

She smiled at my quick protest.

Perhaps she believed, just as childhood specialist Jean Piaget did, that everyone needs to figure out their own successful program. "Every time we teach a child something, we keep him from inventing it himself."—Piaget.

Deadly Serious Tasks.

"I want you to monitor your blood sugar levels often, not just when you get up. Four or five times a day, especially two hours after you eat."

"That's hard to do if you work full-time." I could see me whipping out a glucometer at a meeting to take a blood sugar reading. While everyone watched, I'd prick my finger letting a drop of blood drip onto the lighted strip. Or, I'd lurk in bathrooms to get a fix on my blood sugar.

"It's not hard if you really want to get control of your diabetes."

I didn't have an answer for that one.

"I also want you to stop eating fast food lunches, donuts, and ice cream."

That's the penalty for being honest.

"Pack healthy lunches and snacks."

No more Delicious Sundae Treats.

She then asked, "How will you reward yourself with the money you'll save by bringing food from home?"

"Dinner out at a five star restaurant." Pop! It was out of my mouth with no chance of reeling it back in.

Dr. Carey sighed. "Maybe you could come up with a non-food reward. Rewarding yourself with food is never a good idea."

I didn't protest that food itself had always been a reward for me or that I adored cheeseburgers, fries, and milkshakes. *Me? Pack a lunch? I was beyond lunch box days now that my kids were raised. I was finished with that chore, or so I'd thought.*

Scanning her office for a lunch box, I saw an insulated tote bag. *Man. I couldn't nail her on anything. She's thin. Packs a lunch. She does as she prescribes.*

Drifting thoughts of acquiring a pink, Miss Piggy lunch box were abandoned by the good doctor's next words. Rewards and food diary aside, she cut to the bottom line.

"Your diabetes is out-of-control." She locked her eyes onto mine. "Your vision is already threatened with glaucoma. Your limbs will be affected next. You are running out of oral medications to take. Pills alone can't do it."

Deadly Sweet Tooth.

"Lose weight and exercise. The exercise won't cause you to lose weight, but a twenty-minute walk is as effective as popping a diabetic pill. The blood sugar will be forced into the muscles and burned off. Weight comes off by eating right." She paused and asked, "When will you walk?"

"After work."

"It's more likely to happen if you walk before work or even over your lunch hour."

I could feel rebellion swelling, threatening to overflow, so I switched topics. "The metformin often gives me diarrhea."

"You need that medication unless you want to go on insulin right away."

"I'll learn to live with it."

She ordered more lab work and closed with, "See you in thirty days." Dr. Carey reminded me of Mom, who'd also been a petite dynamo. Plus she'd never listened to any excuses either, particularly about my weight. She'd always said, "Do you want to end up looking like your grandmother?" I didn't have an answer for that one.

The question facing me that I did need to examine was, "Why had I'd gotten derailed and sent to this no-nonsense specialist?" I'd had my type 2 diabetes under control and rewarded myself with a trip to Vegas. *After all, my internist had said I was going to be one of the lucky ones.* How could Vegas be a problem? I'd lost three more pounds there. Actually, I'd gained back twelve pounds rather than the nine my doctors had recorded. My backslide had started after Vegas.

Vegas was not the issue. I hadn't even wanted to come home. How crazy was that? I was a happily married woman, with grown children, and a solid career. Wasn't I? So why did I still want to be in Vegas? Why this big twelve-pound weight gain?

How about—Dreams Spell Trouble?

Part One

Second Chances in Vegas
In the Garden of the Enigma

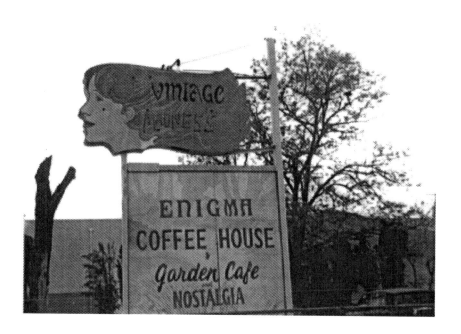

" If nothing ever changed, there would be no butterflies. "
—Unknown

Chapter One...Why VEGAS?

My Vegas vacation almost didn't happen but that wouldn't have been unusual. I've read that 44% of Americans cut their trip short last year, 56% postponed their vacation, 12% skipped their vacation entirely, and 20% felt guilty about taking time off. I didn't feel guilty about taking time off, but my husband knew how to push my guilt button.

"Who'd ever want to go there?" He looked at me from over a library book that he was reading, "What a waste of money."

Complaining to my buddy, Marilyn, that Andy wouldn't even consider Vegas, she said, "Let's do a girlfriend's week."

We made plans and I started packing. A week before departure, Marilyn phoned apologetic.

"I can't go. My boss has given me a killer assignment that has to be done in three weeks or else," said Marilyn. "After that my calendar gets crazy. Maybe we could go in July."

"Going to the desert in July isn't appealing to me."

"I hate letting you down. I know how much you want to see Vegas."

"It's okay," I said, though it wasn't. Trying to be a good sport, I jested, "Vegas is just not in the cards this year."

"I told you I couldn't play cards, anyway. Although, I've been watching Texas Hold-Em on television." Marilyn paused on her cell phone and asked, "Do you want to go to lunch next week?"

"Sure. Why not?"

Grumbling to myself, I set off on my daily hike down Hogsback Lane and up Stinchcomb Hill in the Cleveland Metroparks. The valley below was abandoned by color. Varying hues of mud were the palette of the day, matching my mood. The tail end of February, it had rained four days in a row. No blue relief stretched overhead. Instead, the sky was covered with snotty clouds. Certainly Vegas would have hosted a platter of warm, blue skies.

It didn't matter that under all the beige compost, the land was renewing itself. I wanted spring now. The Rocky River flowing through the valley below was swollen, shredding trees, and other debris in its rush to Lake Erie to empty itself of winter's excess. Inner currents churned, grinding like razors and the resulting muck threatened to spill over and litter the land with tossed stones and silt. Like that river, my body was also swollen with debris. Not only matronly in appearance, I felt old. I was fading to beige trying to meet my mid-life challenges: being my parents' caregiver, paying off our sons' college tuitions, and making all the ends meet. I, too, was seething and struggling to not spill over my banks, out-of-control.

If anyone deserved a reward and a week of room service, it was I. After all, in the nine months since my diagnosis, I'd lost twenty-five pounds. I'd restricted my diet. I'd walked daily. I was beating type 2 diabetes. Plus, as manager of a child welfare agency, my productive region had doubled in size and split in two. Another regional director had been added to supervise the case managers located in three adjacent counties. I had some breathing space. Why not take advantage of it?

Torn, I considered alternatives. I could change my airline ticket and visit family in sunny Florida. I could take the week off and clean my house. Have lunch with friends. Or, I could put on work blinders saving my vacation days for another time. I groaned. *Fat chance of that happening this year.*

Trudging along, a question emerged and ambushed me. *Why not go to Vegas by myself? My bags were packed. And, my calendar was cleared.*

What better place for a person with obvious food and work addictions to go? After all, wasn't it the addiction capital of the world?

Before reaching mid-life, pompous me wouldn't have appreciated Las Vegas. I had viewed Vegas as sleazy with screwed up values. Now I longed for the glitter, the glitz, the gambling frenzy fueled by tattered shreds of hope. It matched the churning inside of me. I wanted to be a free spirit stepping out of character to find new reflections of me. It wasn't that I expected to find myself in Vegas. I didn't want to be found out. What better place for a relief inning or to play a game of hide n' seek!

That's it. Hide n' seek. Now you see Carole. Now you don't. Why don't I go to Vegas by myself? This thought took hold, growing as powerful as the flooding Rocky River. Nothing could stop me from having a great vacation.

My husband and several friends tried to discourage me.

"Vegas? By yourself? Whatever for?"

"You're going through the menopausal crazies."

"Instead, why not buy a red convertible?"

"It's not you."

What was it about me that made Vegas off limits? Did everyone just see me as ancient, sensible?

The travel agent joined the chorus. "Wouldn't a condo by the beach or a cabin in the mountains be more enjoyable?" I could hear her thinking, *More suitable.*

"Look. It's Vegas and that's that," my stubborn nature kicked in. I'd prove them all wrong. "Please arrange for my double occupancy package to be converted into a single."

"Well, since you don't have anyone to split the cost, it'll be expensive. But I'll do my best. And you're right. Everyone should see Vegas at least once, even if all alone."

That's how I found myself in a strange hotel room on the twenty-third floor looking out into the sky overlooking The Strip. The travel agent had done well by me. How my Grandmother Thuresson would have loved the view. She hated and refused to live in ground floor apartments. She always said, "I'm a second story woman."

"Look, Grandmother. I can see the mountains." I hadn't talked or thought to my deceased Grandmother in years, but I found myself doing so.

"Look, over there at the white columns of Caesar's Palace and The Forum. Have you ever seen so many Christmas lights on one street? No wonder it's known as 'The Strip.' It strips away the ordinary and shouts the presence of goodies up and down Las Vegas Boulevard." Sitting at this window would have given Grandmother and me endless hours to spin fairy tales.

Enchanted by the view, I ordered a chicken dinner from room service while watching the day turn into night high above The Strip from my room-side seat. The sky's sunset fought with the lights of The Strip. The sky won, but then retired to leave the night to a billion man-made lights.

A spontaneous cloudburst of tears appeared upon my face. Why the tears? Was it because I couldn't remember the last time I'd watched a sunset? Or, was it because all the lights reminded me of Kathy, my college roommate from South Dakota. She had always loved city lights saying, "I'm a city girl now." Kathy had died six months ago of cervical cancer.

There was a knock at the door. "Room service."

I patted my face with tissue and opened the door. The attendant took one look and asked, "Is everything all right?"

"Yes," I murmured, thinking he probably thought, *This one's only been in Vegas for an hour and has already lost her life's savings.*

He set the table, uncovered the food, and asked, "Would you like the television on for company?"

I tipped him well for his courteous concern.

As soon as he left, I turned off the chatter of the TV and stared at my food. A mammoth baked potato big enough for two and a split chicken breast, black-striped from the grill, lay before me shaped like a broken heart on a platter,

That's me all right, black-striped, heart condition.

I was still angry with my husband for refusing to join me on this trip. When I was dressed and ready to leave, he'd tossed me a square, white box.

"What's this?"

"This is the credit charge you asked me about."

Untying the red ribbon and lifting the lid, a flat pewter pin emerged with a primitive cat drawing engraved upon it. Of all the times to be sentimental! Just when I'd been feeling less than charitable towards him. Had he chosen the cat because we both love cats and usually have a well loved cat or two near us? The pin was labeled, "Kind-Hearted Woman," and the legend inside read:

"When hobos were common to the American experience, they had a vocabulary of hobo signs, chalked or scratched on pavements or fence posts in front of houses to advise or warn off those who might follow. 'Kind-Hearted Woman' is my favorite and describes so many of my friends..."—From Lona Gayst of Drum-Roll Productions.

A lovely gift for the steadfast woman I've tried hard to be, but I wanted more now. Why was it that I yearned... for more, and more of what? I'd pinned the cat on, kissed my husband good-bye, and left for my Vegas vacation. Our grown sons had also given me a going-away gift, the video, *E.T Come Home.* Maybe I needed to run away and act out of character more often. Or, had they sensed and feared something in me that I wasn't aware of yet?

I wasn't particularly hungry. But being diabetic, regular meal times are essential, so I picked at my black-striped, heart dinner before leisurely dressing for a Vegas show. Preening before the mirror, I dabbed a little Bodacious perfume behind my ears.

As I entered the lobby on the swish of high heels and long earrings dangling, a lovely gentleman turned to look at me a second time. When was the last time someone had taken a second look and smiled?

Maybe I ought to go to the theatre more often. With my solo ticket in hand, I was seated as the extra at a table of three friends. No concert rows here. Vegas was forced intimacy at round tables with an attentive bar keep.

"Have a chocolate martini with us, Carole."

"Not right now, but let me buy you a round."

"You shouldn't, but all right," said Sandy the blonde. "We had these at a Christmas lunch and never made it back to work."

Cindy winked and said, "Do you remember those cute guys who bought us round after round?"

"Do I ever," said Sandy. Laughter followed.

"Maybe we can find some of that action here."

More inside jokes about encounters with men followed. I smiled and laughed with them, but couldn't wait for the show to start and then be over to escape this trio who were on a manhunt in Vegas. *This theatrical, Vegas nightlife was not for a solo Carole because it made me feel out of place. Abandoned. Odd woman out. Old.*

After the show, I wished my tablemates luck and escaped to the slot machines. They proved addictive. Reluctantly, I took my meager silver dollar winnings and called gambling quits for the night. The game rooms made me edgy, even though I was still ahead. I'd been further ahead if I'd quit sooner. I hadn't traveled to Vegas to throw my money away to the Vice-Lords of the Strip. I'd come to laugh, have fun, frolic under the lights. *Why did I ever think solitary me would have fun here? What fun?*

Some fun, I thought ignoring the human Keno calling birds while sipping coffee and trashing my Vegas vacation in a windowless, hotel deli. Well, I was here all right, all dressed up, and feeling miserable because Vegas seemed to be for couples or groups of friends. Wallowing in a first class, pity party, I grew angry...finally at the right person... myself.

Why am I feeling sorry for myself? I'm a resourceful person. Surely I could find some fun things to do in Vegas! And if nothing else, the on-call cell phone isn't clipped to my waistband. I'm able to do what I want, when I want, without interruptions. This is my time.

I grabbed a pencil and wrote on a napkin the things that I like and never have time to do. I put a few dreams down and circled one of them, laughing to myself.

By the time my Vegas week was over, I wasn't an E.T. longing for home, but one of the few Americans who thoroughly enjoyed her vacation. However, I was one of the vacation study's 20% who felt guilty. But guilty about what?

For spending money on myself? Why would treating myself to room service and acting on a dream make me feel guilty?

The social worker inside said, *You know why. Who do you think you are splurging hard-earned money on bratty wants, when what you need is four new tires on your car?*

I answered that social worker. *I refuse to become boring, predictable, and an old biddy.*

"What we play is life."
—Louis Armstrong

Chapter Two...Sightseeing in the Garden of the Enigma

Palm trees swayed overhead while patches of snapdragons and full-faced pansies danced along the path leading to three pools linked together with ornamental bridges. Since no one was up and in bikinis at six, I had no reason to be self-conscious about my "no waistline" figure. Fearlessly, I shed my robe and plunged into the middle pool. The desert air and pool were shockingly cold. A feeling of moving through liquid velvet coursed through me as I began swimming laps. My body warmed quickly, from the inside out, as the sun rose over a hushed Vegas.

The only sounds were the attendant's flip-flops as he readied the pool area for the day ahead. He left the lounge chairs facing the west, the pool's auditorium for sun worshipers still asleep in their rooms.

The pool itself was mine and mine alone for this first hour of daylight. What a delicious way to start a February day. Yesterday in Ohio, it had snowed six inches. Dropping off my wet towels at the cabana, I heard the attendant (who looked like a candidate for Mr. Universe), ask, "Are you from Alaska? How can you swim in such cold water?"

"I'm from Ohio, the home of the Cleveland Browns. We never mind a little cold because it knocks out some of the competition."

"That explains it," he said. "Have a good day, Lady Cleveland."

I wondered if the chocolate martini trio had discovered Mr. Universe yet?

Entering the hotel lobby, vacuums and a few diehard pulls of the slot machines were heard from distant gaming rooms. A maid was scrubbing the hallway floor. My wet sandals were leaving definite tracks across the tiles.

"I'm so sorry. Is there another way to reach the elevators?" Guests obviously weren't expected to be swimming so early, but I planned to swim every day of my vacation. It was on my list of favorite things.

"No apology needed," she said arching her back into a big stretch. "There isn't another way to the elevators."

"But your floor's ruined."

"I call that job security." She smiled at me and it was contagious. I chuckled.

Job security, indeed. Point of view was everything.

Back in my room, I headed into the multi-mirrored bathroom. Everyone, everywhere was on display in Vegas, the city of lights, sequins, and mirrors. I pricked my finger and squeezed a drop of blood on the glucometer strip for a blood sugar check. *92. A good reading.* Showered and dressed, I ordered oatmeal and fresh blueberries from room service while checking the yellow pages in the phone book. This Vegas day would be a present to myself. I could feel my excitement growing. I was going live out my all-time, favorite fantasy career. *Drum roll, please, Carole Ingraham Calladine, Globe-Trotting Photo-journalist.*

At the airport yesterday, I had snagged a writers' magazine and honed in on an article on travel writing. Reading it, I learned sales are often tripled when photos accompany the article. Plus, photos document street signs and names. The author devoted a sidebar on how to use a point and shoot camera for dummies. Forget about shutter speeds and *f*-stops. Supposedly, an amateur like me could shoot great pictures as these 35-mm cameras adjusted themselves to light and speed conditions. What I'd previously planned to spend on Vegas revues would be invested in a camera instead.

Catching a bus on The Strip, I transferred to another traveling east on Sahara Avenue and found the full service camera shop that had been listed in the yellow pages. An hour later, I had six rolls of film and my first new camera since the Brownie box camera of my childhood.

Next to the camera store was a stationery shop. I lingered another hour there before choosing a blank journal with a paisley cover and a smooth flowing pen with blue ink. What fun to write myself in streams of blue. This was a welcome change from the black ink mandated for charting psychosocials, measurable social work goals, and counseling interventions.

Pleased with my purchases, I set off to find one of the forty plus chapels that dot the Vegas landscape. One of the spunky case managers that I supervised wanted a wedding chapel postcard for her boyfriend.

"He's always saying, 'Let's run away to Vegas and get married.'"

"Do you really want to get married in Vegas?"

"I just want to marry him. I'll send the postcard with just one word on it. Yes."

I wondered how many other couples seriously considered skipping off to Vegas. There might be a story here. I found and shot the wedding chapel that proclaimed that Michael Jordan and Joan Crawford had been married within. I assumed they were never married to each other, but you couldn't tell it by the sign. Giggling, I ducked inside and asked for a postcard for a back-up image, in case even a camera for dummies was beyond me.

Handing me a postcard, the attendant asked, "For yourself? A daughter?"

"Not for me, and I don't have a daughter," I laughed. "But, where is the marriage license bureau?"

At the intersection of Third and Carson in downtown Vegas, couples were departing from trucks, modest sedans, and white stretch limos. Climbing the steps with them into the Clark County Court House, I was amazed that the marriage license bureau hosted a full house on a weekday morning. The bureau's hours were: "M—Th: 8 AM till Midnight, Friday: 8AM till Sunday at Midnight."

As a wannabe journalist, I joined a line of couples seeking to talk to one of the four clerks. When my turn came, a middle-aged clerk peered around me and asked, "Where's the other half of your couple?"

"At home, in Ohio." *Besides, I didn't want a marriage license. Maybe a divorce decree, but not a marriage license.*

"A friend asked me to get some Vegas marriage information."

"Likely story," she said giving me the once over. She handed me an information sheet and a blank application shooing me away, saying, "Next, please."

Such rudeness. Did she get a commission on how many licenses that she processed in an hour?

The application consisted of seventeen questions.No legal documents were required such as a birth certificate or divorce decree. The processing fee was $35 and the stamped marriage license was good for one year. What could be easier?

Signs on the walls warned widows and widowers that their social security benefits might be affected by getting married. The female could completely lose hers if she only qualified under her deceased husband's benefits. A posted newspaper article explained why it is more economical to live in sin after sixty. Guess there's still plenty of marrying going on after age 65. *Hmm. Another story?*

A salesman arrived with flyers advertising wedding bouquets and was efficiently escorted to the door by a guard. I went over to the guard and asked, "Does this happen often?"

"It usually only happens once because everyone knows that we enforce the no solicitation policy. But hey, they're just trying to make a buck."

At last, someone in the know was willing to talk to me. "What does it cost to get married in Vegas?"

"Well now, the local justice of the peace charges $35 for a wedding ceremony. They're across the street in the Bridger Building."

"Not bad. Sure beats the cost of most weddings."

"Marriage is a booming industry here. Over seventy thousand couples get married in Vegas every year." He shifted his considerable weight and asked, " So are you thinking about getting married here?"

I flashed my wedding band and said, "Already married."

"Some couples come to renew their vows and have a second honeymoon."

"My husband thinks Vegas is a waste of money."

The guard shook his head at me. "He's letting a pretty thing like you walk around all alone?"

Flattered, I laughed. "Yes, he is."

Outside, I followed a young couple who was heading straight for the Bridger Building. Inside the front door, the color red was everywhere –red walls, red carpet, red seat cushions. The lobby screamed red. Someone took the poetic line literally: "My love is like a red, red rose." Then again, some ironic decorator might be saying, "Stop. Think about what you're doing here."

Another marriage option was available at this intersection. Across the street stood The First United Methodist Church and Chapel. I wanted to investigate, but I found the doors locked. The Church was obviously not soliciting for weddings despite its ideal location. A stone marker proclaimed this to be the oldest church in Las Vegas founded by Reverend W. Bain, Pastor, on June 18, 1905. Engraved on this marker was a scripture.

"Your old men shall dream dreams. Your young men shall see visions." Joel: 2:28

Now that I was age 50, I was standing at the crossroads. In-between young and old, was I a dreamer, or a visionary? Could I be both? This paradoxical message resonated within.

Lots to think about. Fifty is quite a milestone. I had received a birthday card that read: Fifty is the old age of youth and the youth of old age.

Thus preoccupied and wandering on Fourth Street, I saw a carved, brown bear standing on its hind legs. *A bear? In the middle of the desert? Why not a horse or a camel?* (Later, I learned that bears are a Native American symbol for strength and healing.) I only knew that I was drawn to the bear that seemed in and out of place at the same time in the middle of old Las Vegas.

While taking Mr. Bear's picture, I thought, *perhaps he and Goldilocks had temporarily reversed roles. Goldilocks. Of course. That was my immediate connection to Mr. Bear. I was Goldilocks looking for "just the right experience" in a town that had it all. Goldilocks had eaten the "just the right porridge" and fell asleep in a "just the right bed" only to be awakened from her dreams and chased home. I wondered if Goldilocks ever ventured forth in the woods again? And what was Goldilocks really doing wandering alone in the woods in the first place? Maybe a girl of any age needed to venture forth alone while finding her "just right" self.*

Further down on Fourth Street, a sign announced the "Enigma, Garden Cafe and Nostalgia." The words were irresistible even though the place looked like a closed relic of the past. It couldn't possibly be a thriving business. I snapped documentation shots with my new camera before venturing down the weed-cracked driveway.

Tucked away behind this weathered century house in Vegas, was a garden haven frequented by the locals. Hot tea was being served and I had some while reading area newspapers, eavesdropping, and viewing art offerings by a native artist, Magda Szeitz. Ms. Szeitz recovered rectangular molding pieces from an architectural salvage company, pieced them together, and painted in the spaces created. Finished pieces were similar to icons decorated with various figures and beadwork. *Was Ms. Szeitz a visionary or a dreamer thinking she could make something out of salvage? I thought, She's probably both. That's what happens when one is creative. One becomes ageless.*

Lingering, I behaved myself ordering a pita pocket stuffed with veggies and sprouts for lunch. I knew then that no matter what, Vegas would be a satisfying vacation. How rejuvenating to swim at dawn and lounge in gardens in February. Unlike Goldilocks, I found a "just right" spot without disapproving bears making me feel obsolete by brushing me aside and saying, "You must have a chocolate martini." Or, "Next, please."

Inhaling desert sunshine and blue sky, I watched long tailed birds flit in birdbaths. Blue ink pen in hand, I began to write about my day. "How had I found the perfect experience in Vegas that I was seeking without even knowing it?"

Now where had I heard that sentiment expressed before? Writing the question out, I remembered. It came to me as a gift, appropriately so, as it had been connected with gift giving.

When our son, Brendan, was approaching his tenth birthday, he said, "I don't know what I want." He thought some more and said, "I have ice skates, a baseball mitt, and a bike. But, a birthday is a birthday." He shrugged his shoulders, smiled at his father and me. "You'll think of something."

A few days later, Andy, my husband and expert child detective, suggested, "How about a camera? He's responsible and old enough to look after it."

Because this would be Brendan's entire birthday gift, I held my breath as he tore off the paper. He carefully lifted the camera out of the box. Even his eyes smiled up at us. "How did you know what I wanted when I didn't know it myself?"

Exactly right, Brendan. How did I know what's wanted when I didn't even know it myself? Yet today, on the very first day of my Vegas vacation, I'd found a 35-mm camera, snagged a blank journal, explored the Vegas marriage phenomenon, discovered the "Enigma," marveled at beaded icons made from salvaged moldings, and was intrigued with the lingering question of whether I was young or old, a dreamer or visionary. Playing at being a travel writer and gathering facts about my surroundings amused me.

While writing, more and more scattered thoughts kept intruding. As a counselor I'd learned how to be quiet and focused. I was the listener of other people's challenges and not the teller of my own. *Why was it that I didn't extend the courtesy of being heard to myself?*

At a table in the Enigma, I did listen and journaled about being a social worker where building connections to troubled strangers and hearing their life traumas had given my life purpose but had also worn me down. After my mom died, I closed my flourishing family counseling office to work regular nine-to-five hours in an agency in order to spend more time with my grieving Dad. Did I really believe that I'd only work nine-to-five? And after a few months of seeing my dad daily, he left me. Traveling south, he joined his fellow snowbirds for the winter. Nothing had really changed, yet everything had.

I'd returned to my child welfare roots as a regional director, supervising new social workers, listening second-hand to the life traumas of neglected and abused children and their families. Maybe my career shift had more to do with my wanting to be an earth mother, to make up for the loss and ache that I was feeling rather than facing it head on. When Mom died, I felt orphaned. An unexpected shock. Did everyone feel this way, regardless of age, when a mother died?

Even though Mom and I had our differences, she was there for me and I for her. She took her last breath on my watch while I read her favorite poem, *I Wandered Lonely as a Cloud,* that concludes –

"For oft, when on my couch I lie
In vacant or in pensive mood,
They flash upon that inward eye
Which is the bliss of solitude;
And then my heart with pleasure fills,
And dances with the daffodils."
—William Wordsworth

I whispered into the paisley journal, *"I know you found the host of golden daffodils, Mom."* The tears came and I didn't try to stop them even if I could have. I was amongst strangers in the Garden of the Enigma. My tears, like a fine spring rain, cleansed me inside out. Some fell on the page and blurred the daffodils.

"Miss you, Mom."

Sipping hot tea in the bliss of solitude, I thought how blessed I'd been to have a mother who fussed over me. She gave me piano lessons, balanced meals, and taught me how to swim.

A memory of an another mother nudged at me, a memory I had blackened out on purpose. *Why was this memory calling to me now? Hell's bells. What's the use? Might as well let it in.*

While on a recent drive with Linda Thayer to Columbus to install her as a board member from the Cleveland region, she and I had been exchanging pleasantries about our families. Then, as it always does when you least want it to ring, the on-call, cell phone clipped to my belt rang.

"This is Carole Calladine."

"This is Marsha from Cuyahoga. We need a foster home for a two- or three-year-old male that the police just brought in."

"Can you tell me more? I have several placements for that age child. What are the child's special needs?"

"We don't even know his name, let alone his needs. The neighbors phoned the police because they heard the child crying and hadn't seen the mom in several days. The police broke in and found him eating paper lying beside his dead mother. Appears to be a drug overdose." Marsha paused and I could hear her talking to her supervisor. "Is Ms. Higgins available? Our computer shows that her foster children went home last week."

"Yes, the Johnson brothers were reunified with their mom last week." I thought, *The sheets are barely cold. Would having another child so soon be in Ms. Higgins's best interests?* "Let me check and see if she's ready to take a child."

I phoned one of our case managers, related the story, and the request for Ms. Higgins.

"I'll take care of it and have a safe journey to Columbus, Carole."

Crisis over, I turned to Linda and said, "You just witnessed what we do."

"How can you be so cold?" asked Linda bursting into tears. "Don't you care?"

I felt that I had been slapped in the face. *"So cold!"... Now don't get defensive, Carole. The uninitiated is shocked by the stories we hear everyday.* I took a deep breath and counted to ten before answering Linda, speaking very softly.

"It's hard to hear the children's stories but it wouldn't do anyone any good if I fell apart, now would it?" I looked over at Linda as she mopped up her tears with a tissue. "And I assure you, I do care or I wouldn't do this work."

By the time we reached Columbus, Linda was committed to the agency's mission and soon became a passionate board member. But her hurtful question remained and picked at my psyche.

"How can you be so cold?"

Now, in the Garden of the Enigma, I had time to ponder Linda's question. I put the question in bold letters on a journal page and set about answering it. I did know how to put on my clinical armor and filter out feelings. How else could one deal with a toddler eating paper lying beside a dead mother or the hundred other family tragedies, such as the screams of an eight-year-old having a bath when a delusional father threw a feral cat in the tub with her?

As an administrator, I clamped these feelings off. But did they drive me to work longer and longer hours magically thinking that there must be an end somewhere? All it succeeded in doing so far was to double the region, which thankfully, had just split in two. I was back to supervising seven rather than fourteen case managers and overseeing services for a hundred rather than two hundred children. Could I work a regular nine-to-five schedule now? Or, had I only raised the bar of possible daily expectations the staff? Would we soon be recruiting thirty new foster families and supervising 200 again?

It's no wonder the staff and I fantasized about taking *fun* vacations on stressful days because social work is never a job that can be left at the office. Or, we'd fantasize about taking no-brainer jobs. My favorite was selling tickets in an afternoon theater kiosk surrounded by the smell of buttery popcorn and promises of *happily ever after* screen stories.

Or, maybe my new favorite could be a travel writer in the tradition of William Hurt in *The Accidental Tourist.* I'd teach lone women travelers how to carry a book and mumble incoherently to themselves to discourage unwanted conversations. Reviewing pleasing accommodations and meals was a cake job. I'd be good at the cake and meal part. (Finally I was laughing at myself.) Or, perhaps I could clean Vegas hotel lobbies at night polishing the floors that would be scuffed and marked by the following evening. Wouldn't that be better than seeing one more hurt child or disturbed parent who had never had a lioness mom like I'd had to protect them?

Someone had to protect the children and help their families. I was good at it because I could detach myself from what had happened and see what needed to be done for healing to occur. Perhaps Linda's question bothered me for other reasons. *Were the multiple children and their families becoming my phantom life? How long could I do this work without permanently shutting down feelings? Or, had I already shut down my feelings?*

But enough, enough already. These ideas were too hard on such a beautiful vacation day. *What was this? A vacation or an extreme makeover?* I had no new vision of myself, other than being a social worker. I was proud of my profession. Wasn't I just spending a week dreaming dreams, playing, and getting away from it all?

Just taking a break from real life, Ma'am, just a break. Close your journal. Smile for the camera. Click. That's how I ended up tear-stained, limp, yet frozen in place on the first day of my vacation in the Garden of the "Enigma" with a giant question mark planted in my chest. It was in my best interests that I forgot a counseling truism that the mind has to play awhile before it can take in new ideas that challenge routines and beliefs. If I'd remembered, I'd have run scared, back to the hotel, and caught the first plane home immersing myself in my old life before it was too late to do so.

*"Every blade of grass has its Angel that bends over it
and whispers, 'Grow, grow.'"*
—The Talmud

Chapter Three...Life's Buffets & the Little Girl's Room

Everyone from my airline seatmates to the room service attendant said, "Don't miss the buffet at Caesar's Palace." Plus, as a photo-journalist, I needed to add some Vegas eateries to my repertoire.

I stood in the doorway of the Palace buffet and peeked in. Lush flower arrangements, lit ice sculptures, and tables loaded with inviting food, stretched as far as the eye could see. Buttery bakery smells reached out and wrapped themselves around me. "Do you have a reservation?" asked the hostess, a Suzanne Somers's look-alike.

I managed to clear my throat, gulp, and croak, "No."

"A table for one?"

I nodded.

"Follow me."

So I did. The long-legged hostess headed deep into an immaculate, white linen dining room where attentive waiters filled wineglasses and removed plates of half-eaten food. The patrons boasted about choice morsels, going back for seconds. Everywhere, food sirens assaulted me, and I found myself as Pavlov's dog drooling on cue. My body literally trembled. Growing more anxious by the mini-second, I thought, *I could get into serious, big mouth trouble here.*

As the hostess pulled out a chair to seat me at a remote table by the swinging kitchen door, I balked and said, "I'm not hungry enough to do justice to this feast."

Then I marched myself out of that buffet room on my short legs, head held high, without looking to the left or to the right, focused on the blessed doorway. Once outside Caesar's Palace, my feet flew to the bus stop. While riding the bus to the closest intersection to the Enigma, I snagged my last apple out of my backpack. Slowly, I ate this apple not caring that its juices ran down my chin. I felt my taste buds and stomach settle down.

Ever since a commute from Cleveland to Columbus, Ohio for the monthly state management meeting, I've carried an apple as part of my survival kit. I'd have to remember to find some more apples today or I could even have a fruit basket delivered to my room to replenish my supply while in Vegas.

Feeling calmer, I entered the Garden of the Enigma and ordered a tuna salad wrap and a pot of rose hip tea. I savored each sip and bite. Feeling pleased with myself for choosing the right repast, I knew it was time to explore in my journal the interrelated topics of diabetes, buffets, and the little girl's rooms.

I never wanted to forget how I ended up stuck in each rest stop visiting the little girl's room along Interstate 71, between Columbus and Cleveland. The day had started wrong. I'd overslept and flown through my usual morning routine squeezing in a brief exercise tape and shower before driving with a lead foot to agency headquarters in Columbus. On the way, I picked up a fast food breakfast at the gas station. Munching along the highway, a round of sausage buckshot had stained my blouse. Then the remains of this sandwich eaten on the run had sat in my stomach feeling like a cannonball ready to explode. I'd hoped a sane lunch of salad greens would neutralize my distress. No such luck.

"We've ordered in pizza to save money and time today," announced the boss.

I groaned inside. I should have skipped lunch, but I wanted to be a good sport and appear normal, as only my family knew about my diabetes. I nibbled at a wedge of plain cheese pizza.

"Come on, Carole. Help us finish up."

"Have a second slice. You've lost enough weight."

"Everyone else has eaten two or more except you, Carole."

So I did. I had seconds taking the last piece of pizza. This time seconds was more than my poor digestive system could handle. I felt the pepperoni & cheese combo jump upon and ignite the breakfast cannonball that resided in my stomach. Ka-boom! Diarrhea plagued me for the next seven hours.

Driving home, I was in agony and reduced to stopping at all the rest areas yearning to be at home, in my own bathroom. I lectured myself endlessly at every exit. I should've taken time to eat a bowl of cereal at the kitchen table, braved the heat for arriving late, skipped my exercise tape, not had a second piece of pizza. Maybe, I should check myself into a motel for a private bathroom, or follow the hospital road signs asking for an enema in the emergency room. Or, I could just shoot myself and put myself out of my misery. Somehow, I arrived home five hours later, two hours longer than usual.

I died for another hour in my own bathroom followed by a tub soak relaxing my shaken body whose surface felt clammy to the touch. Blood sugar of 280 plus was raging war in my body. Andy hovered outside the bathroom door.

"What can I do to help you?"

"I ate wrong and I don't want to talk about it."

He knew enough to not say more. I fixed myself a bowl of chicken soup and took a diabetic pill while he cheerfully ate a bowl of cereal with skim milk and two pieces of whole wheat toast for dinner.

The next morning, I wondered if this was what an alcoholic felt like coming off a binge. I was shaky inside. Even my bones felt swollen and wobbly. My botchy skin felt and smelled like a piece of overripe fruit.

Two days later while visiting with a friend, she asked how my week had been. I confided in her about my "fast food," Columbus commute from hell. She confided a similar experience at a college reunion party after a rich dinner of chicken divan. We gossiped about a friend who had to change at the wedding reception from her beautiful, ice pink, "Mother of the Groom" dress because of a sudden onslaught of uncontrollable diarrhea.

I laughed and said, "When we were young mothers, we were preoccupied with our babies' bowel movements. Are we going to start this talk again as 'women of a certain age' movements?"

My friend remained serious despite my laughter. "No one talks about this, Carole. But when the taboo is broken, women are eager to talk. I've discovered most women think they are the only ones."

"Aging bodies and failing bowels. All this talk has made me think that maybe a box of adult diapers is needed for special occasions."

But my friend wasn't laughing. Instead she was thinking about purchasing some as a precaution.

To myself I thought, *I had only been kidding, hadn't I?*

Writing in my paisley Vegas journal, I could no longer kid myself. I must rid myself of "no time to eat right" stresses and greasy, "fast food" backslides. Then surely I would have a few, good digestible years left. Eating right and slowing down would prevent getting stuck in the *little girl's room. Little Girl's Room*, indeed! Getting stuck in the *Old Girls' Room* was more like it.

In adolescence, I had toyed with making the *little girls' room* my lifelong friend in staying skinny while eating with reckless abandon. The Homecoming Queen, Bridget Nelson, inadvertently let me in on her lunchtime secret.

Bridget held court in the cafeteria eating chips and ice cream. I could only dream of eating a shiny bag of potato chips or an ice-cream bar. Cafeteria lunches were regimented eating times for me. My mom was the high school cafeteria manager. I ate the "special" whether I liked it or not. The boys proclaimed Mom a wonderful cook. Many confided that the cafeteria lunches were better than their mother's dinners.

There's no doubt about it. Mom could have organized a full-scale, gourmet mess for an army. Efficient in her trim, white nylon uniform, she paid attention to what her teen clientele liked and what was healthy.

Eating the daily special, I watched the ebb and flow of social interactions as intense as the ocean's ever-present undercurrent. However, the one lunch room scene that I remember the most, didn't occur in the cafeteria. It occurred in the *little girls' room*, down a quiet hallway, off the gym. I'd made a dash to this rest room, as the one off the cafeteria had been jammed. I didn't want to be late to class. From the end stall, I could hear someone retching. Washing my hands, I debated whether to help the sick student to the nurse's office. Another student, who'd come in to put on cherry red lipstick whispered, "Don't look so worried. This happens every day. She forces herself to lose her lunch."

I felt my eyes registering shock and my mouth went mute. Bridget Nelson, the Homecoming Queen, emerged from the end stall. She chose a sink, gargled some mouthwash, and brushed her damp curly hair into place.

Bridget had entered public high school after graduating from the town's K-8, parochial school. With her innocent beauty and good manners, she was worshipped by the underclassmen. Formerly, she had been my favorite librarian assistant in the children's room at the Clinton Public Library. There she had acted kindly to me, a principal's daughter who was four years younger and a bookworm with thick-lensed glasses. She'd chatted regularly with me. But when I entered high school, we only nodded in passing. She had changed and I knew that I was a reminder of how she once looked.

At the library, she'd been a plump tomato, not unlike my maternal grandmother. Now Bridget was hourglass curvy with a tiny waist. She was a butterfly who had shed her formerly squishy body. Despite her first blush of redness upon seeing me in the rest room, she resumed her serene countenance and smiled at me as if nothing unusual had happened.

I didn't ask if she was okay. This was unmentionable. Dazed from this encounter, I was ten minutes late for biology class and received a detention. But it had been worth it because Oprah and Dr. Phil weren't around then and bulimia was not a common act. I'd learned the secret of how the butterfly had emerged. And, I was envious. The Homecoming Queen knew how to eat her cake and suffer no weighty consequences.

A few weeks later at the Blackhawk Hotel's Sunday Buffet, I stuffed myself and ended the feast with two of the world's best chocolate eclairs despite Mom's glare. Then I excused myself to use the *little girl's room.* I stuck my finger down my throat; gagged, perspired, but couldn't vomit. Throwing up at will was a skill that was obviously beyond me. Instead my stomach groaned and popped out like a balloon. I was miserable and knew that I'd never be a Homecoming Queen.

I'd tucked that long ago scene in some compartment of my brain not wanting to think about it. But now that I'd written it down in my journal, I couldn't escape the stomach burdens that I took to the *little girl's room.* Nor could I escape how I'd been using food. Its use wasn't for nourishment. Rather, food and thoughts of food plagued me. Even made me ill. A deep sense of shame enveloped me. Shame for all the excessive chocolate éclair choices that I'd made over and over again just because it tasted good.

If I didn't permanently reform myself, I was going to wear shame as a shroud and the *old girl's room* was going to be my aging body's destination right along with a needle and insulin. I needed to stick to eating just enough to make my body hum. I needed to pass on any buffet. After all, I was diabetic now. Diabetes in some medical circles was known as the "hoof-and-mouth" disease. Translated, that meant too little exercise and too much food. That had been me all right. I'd take a little taste of everything placing it on my plate as an appetizer, then I'd have heaping second portions of my favorites. I was eating enough for two or three people in one sitting. No wonder I'd laughed at the dietician's plastic servings of a regulated, chicken dinner. Ten bites and the meal was over. No wonder I'd gotten fat because my pancreas couldn't produce enough insulin to keep up with me.

Diet and exercise. It sounded so simple, yet it was so hard. Losing the twenty-five pounds pre-Vegas hadn't been easy and I needed to lose twenty-five more and twenty-five more after that. Perhaps I should post a picture of the *little girls' room* on my car visor and refrigerator with the questions, "What's your hurry? What is your true destination? Your grandmother's wide-bottom rocker and the rest-rooms of life?"

Along side this photo, I'd post a saying attributed to Gandhi: "There is more to life than increasing your speed." I needed to slow down. I needed to eat right. I needed to think of *diet*, not as a word of scarcity, but synonymous with another four-letter word that held great meaning for me. That word was *"Life."*

A poem took shape in my mind. I chuckled to myself as the pen flew across the journal page.

Ode to Food

Move over platters of food.
You are no longer
The glittering buffet in my life.
We can be acquaintances, but not
Inseparable companions.
I will not graze anymore.
Instead, I will breathe deeply.
I will feel anxious, sad,
Frustrated, angry,
And even joyful
Without stuffing myself
Comatose by your
Perpetual presence.
I need
S
P
A
C
E
To feel,

Experience
Life
Fully
Unadorned
Without whipped-creamed, chocolate sundae celebrations.
Or, buttered popcorn, potato chip video feasts for unwinding.
Put the hors d'oeuvres, tarts, and petits fours away and...
"But,"
No buts—let me finish, please.
It has taken me forever to confront you.
I love you, yet
You are the devil's trident
Dipped in sweet and salty disguise.
Not good for more than four visits per day.
Count them.
Breakfast. Lunch. Dinner. Snack.
Or,
Breakfast. Dinner. Snack. Supper.
I will visit you four times a day.
No more. No less.
No. You cannot visit me.
I mean what I say.
Too much of you is toxic, unhealthy.
You can no longer be a constant companion.
I'm sorry that you feel abandoned.
I must push away from your tempting smorgasbord.

Throw open the window.
Fill the room with new aromas:
Fresh-cut grass,
Blooming lilacs, marigolds,
Drifting trails of wood-smoke.
I must hike into a lifeline
Of unlimited possibilities.
I will no longer
Live to eat myself silly.
Instead, I will eat
Savoring life itself.

"Evening/ page by page/ I hum beneath my quilt."
—Yu Hsuan-Chi

Chapter Four...My Second Story Grandmother

Pulling the bed sheets taut with hospital corners before going to the Garden of the Enigma, I made my hotel bed instead of leaving it for the maid to do. This bed-making ritual was instilled by my mother and wouldn't wait. I cannot abandon an unmade bed. I've tried but it shocks me to return to such a disheveled bed making me as uncomfortable as the childhood rhyme, "Step on a crack, break your mother's back." Dishes in the sink, strewn newspapers, dust on the buffet, none of these disturb my sense of order in the world, but an unmade bed traps me. The hotel satin coverlet was slippery and hard to center. At home my wedding quilt stitched by my grandmother centers easily and transforms my bed into a glorious garden of flowers. Bleeding hearts, pansies, tulips, morning glories, roses, daffodils, and snapdragons smile and wave at me.

Basking in sunlight at the Enigma savoring a cup of rose hip tea, I opened the paisley journal—my confidant. Before taking in another tourist attraction for my feature story on Vegas, I wanted to write about my grandmother, Amy G. Thuresson. I'd always thought she had a contrary influence on me, but I wasn't so sure after arriving and talking to her constantly in Vegas. *What was that all about?*

I can still see her sitting in her turret window in her double-wide rocker humming a favorite hymn such as, *"He walks with me and He talks with me,"* quilting hoop in her ample lap. At the family party for my twelfth birthday, she gave me the gorgeous flower quilt.

"I can't wait to put it on my bed, Grandma."

"Oh, no. It's not for now," she said, stroking my arm. "This quilt is for a double bed for when you marry."

"Oh!" *Marriage. My mother had never married until she was thirty and that seemed a lifetime away.* "Oh," was the only word I could manage as I gave her a hug and kissed her soft cheek. After we examined each flower framed in green, the wedding quilt was wrapped in a cotton sheet to be put away for safekeeping.

My mother redecorated my bedroom and gave me a second quilt on my twelfth birthday. She'd made a pink and blue, pinwheel quilt on her Singer sewing machine.

Viewing it, grandmother said, "It's very uniform." She paused and then added, "Kind of takes the fun out of quilting, don't you think?"

I looked at my mother who said, "Machine quilting gives me time to do other things, and this quilt is a perfect color match for the new, rose trellis wallpaper in Carole's room." She turned on her heel and said, "Dinner will be ready in a few minutes."

Later that day, my best friend, JeriKay asked, "What did you get for your birthday?"

"Two quilts."

My friend was polite but I could tell she thought, *How boring.*

"I wanted a desk," I said. My earliest dreams were to be a writer. I could tell she didn't think much of that idea for a present either.

As an adult writer seeking nuances of truth, I found the past was a present waiting to be opened and looked at again. Nuggets to be discovered among faulty assumptions. Grandmother had lived on Fifth Avenue in Clinton, Iowa. Her curved window apartment on the second floor jutted out over the entrance of a lumber baron's former mansion. The lumber baron's family had long since taken their profitable stash and left this sedentary Mississippi River town. In my childhood, the town of Clinton was supported by its major industry, Du Pont, maker of cellophane. Wood pulp treated with caustic soda, carbon disulphide and water solidifies into a clear film and created an odor not unlike overripe gym laundry left hanging out to dry. The lumber barons had left their mark, scent, and then run off to more pleasant smelling surroundings.

My grandmother's son, my Uncle Earl, had followed their example and run off, too, making a fortune in the Oregon lumber business leaving Mom behind to take care of their parents. My mother was the dutiful daughter, who'd brought home from college a husband who became the hometown's middle-school principal. She ended up feeling stuck, especially when her complaining mother in her fifties became a widow. I always thought that's why my mother encouraged me to find a future elsewhere. So I ran off to social work graduate school. I now think she'd hoped that I'd land in Chicago, Minneapolis, or even Des Moines and be within an afternoon's driving distance. In the end, she would have to move to Cleveland for me to see her through her final illness.

As a child, I visited Grandmother often. Mom dropped me off every Tuesday to take piano lessons from Mrs. Nickelson who lived behind my grandmother on Fourth Avenue in a squat, six-suite apartment building. Her first floor apartment was made smaller by the dominance of the baby grand piano in the living room. Sitting there, I'd felt squeezed, squeezed into something I could never be, learning the musical scales to a metronome. Tick tock. Tick tock. After a forever hour and free of Mom's planned lessons for the day, I'd skip around the block to grandmother's apartment for a visit.

Elms soared up and down Fifth Avenue, their canopy making this wide street seem grand, unlike the occasional, scrawny tree on Fourth Avenue. The former mansion where grandmother resided was built with no expense spared. The castle proper was square and well proportioned made out of gray field stone and red brick. On its right flank were the former stables, turned into four ground floor apartments. My grandmother wouldn't consider living on the ground level because she loved a view. She'd been so pleased when she'd found this second story apartment with strong northern light. My mother thought the apartment was impractical, but grandmother wouldn't hear her protests. She'd arranged for a mover to cart selected contents from her former home and settled into her eagle's nest. Her windows faced the front doors of Fifth Avenue's First Presbyterian Church, where hymns played on the hour from the bell tower.

Climbing the wide stone steps of the arched front porch, I'd look up to the turret window. My grandmother, the queen, would be waving. No one got in or out without being under her scrutiny. Opening the right side of the carved mahogany, double entrance doors, I'd look up the twenty-four steps of a wide spiral staircase. Grandmother only climbed these steps once a week on Sunday, huffing and puffing, when she went to church followed by dinner at our house. Throughout the rest of the week, everyone came to her. The neighbors even trotted her mail from the vestibule up to her door.

She'd lean on her cane at the top of the staircase waiting and expecting a kiss from me on her proffered cheek. Wisps of gray brown hair framed her face, falling from her rubber-banded bun. She'd refuse mother's offer to have it cut conveniently short, just as she'd refuse mother's frequent entreaties to move her to the Sarah Harding Home, a residence with elevators for the senior ladies of the town.

"What if there is a fire?" Mom asked. "How will you ever get out on time?"

"Life is too short for such worries," Grandmother would reply. "Having a wonderful view and natural light is what's important." And that was that, as she'd then change the subject.

Grabbing my arm, Grandmother and I shuffle-stepped us to her rocker in the cupola windows. A round pedestal table with a tray of purple and pink African violets, centered in the window nook with a companion chair, made an inviting window grouping. Other residents of the building often dropped in to sit, chat, and enjoy the best view in the house.

Parked in her sunlit spot, she'd send me to the kitchen to fetch a plate of Oreos and tall glasses of whole milk. Grandmother liked having someone at her beck and call and was good at giving orders. Besides sweets, she was crazy for sloppy joe's which were always made up in her refrigerator. She knew my love of Oreos would bring me near.

Grandmother weighed lots. How much she weighed, I never knew because her scale didn't go past 250 pounds. So that became her agreed upon weight. She made her housedresses and wore them covered by a full-length, bib apron. Grandmother might have been a type 2 diabetic, but she was never diagnosed as such. Her concern was always her heart, fainting spells, and arthritis. When she complained about these ailments, her daughter said, without sympathy, "You'd feel better if you lost some weight."

Grandmother would order in her preferred groceries and treat the delivery boy to lemonade or hot chocolate depending on the season. Mother brought her fruits and vegetables, but my grandmother confided in me that she only ate the grapes.

"I give the rest away to my neighbors," she'd brag. "Mrs. Webster is partial to the zucchini and makes a wonderful zucchini nut bread. She brings it over still warm from the oven." She'd sigh, wink, and add, "Don't tell your mother."

It seems to me that my grandmother and mother were always in a tug of war over living arrangements, a proper diet, and even over me. Cast as the child spy carrying news between households, I'd quickly learned silence and how to be evasive when questions were asked. Always uncomfortable when both were in the same room, I didn't want to be expected to choose a side, and quickly learned not to do so. (Later these witnessed, conflictual exchanges proved helpful in becoming a counselor.)

A framed photograph of my grandfather as a young man in a dark suit and white shirt sat on the mantle shelf watching over us just as my grandmother watched the outside world. Maybe she felt better up high. Maybe she even felt closer to grandfather in her turret window thrust into the sky. Whatever the reason, she was a real second story woman entering her daily world through an upstairs window.

My earliest memory was of grandfather's death. Mother said that couldn't be possible since I'd been only three. I don't remember him; I remember death. The dining room filled with morning light as the venetian blinds branded shadow stripes across wall and rug. I couldn't be mistaken of what I saw because Mother entered the room crying, and she never cried. Dad was holding her as if she would break in two from her sobs. I was frightened. They weren't aware of my presence, so I crept back to my bedroom, and took comfort, sucking my fingers and rocking myself. Grandmother and I both soothed ourselves by eating and rocking back and forth, back and forth.

Later that day, my brother, John and I were taken next door to Bestamo and Bestafa Juhl's house, our Danish grandparents related by proximity and mutual affection. (Bestamo and my mother were both presidents of the YWCA board during their lifetimes and were given silver tea sets in appreciation for their tireless service.) I now understood that the Juhls provided my mother the extended family she wished for after her adored father died. Plus, Mom blamed Grandmother for her dad's early heart attack. "My mother is so difficult," I heard her confide to a friend. "Always badgering to get her way. I think she wore Dad out."

In grandmother's apartment, a half table hugged the entry wall, opposite the floor to ceiling, built-in bookcase. This cherry table was now in my home. Grandfather had rescued it from a neighbor's bonfire, sawed off the smoldering side, and made a decorative table at my grandmother's suggestion. On it, she'd kept her Bible and a blue china dish with her house keys. Grandmother would always finish the story of the rescued table by saying, "Those McHugh's never had any sense of what was worth saving."

The eating of the ritual Oreos was a big treat. Grandmother didn't mind when I split them open and ate the filling first and then dipped the chocolate wafer into my milk. When she picked up a quilt square, that would be the signal to clear the table before Mother came and caught us eating cookies.

I'd wash and dry the glasses, wipe up the telltale, dark chocolate crumbs, and then take a clean cloth and polish the tabletop until its oak-grained surface gleamed. I'd also polish the pedestal leg and the four, clawed feet as Grandmother's girth preventing her from doing this herself. Grandmother would nod in approval. Next, she'd always want me to work on my tea towel because needlework was her perfected craft, but French knots and petal stitches required more patience then I possessed after school and a piano lesson. I think Grandmother thought the needlework was more important than the piano playing, but she knew to keep silent enjoying our mid-week visits.

"I'll work on it when you come over on Sunday, Grandmother," I'd tell her. "Let me read to us today." Grandmother knew my plan was to be a writer, but reminded me that being married and having children came first. (How early we women are programmed by the women who love us and think they know what's best for us.)

Walking to Grandmother's bookcase filled me with a different kind of pleasure. I'd select a book and curl up in the window chair dangling my legs over its wooden arms without fear of reprimand. Carefully opening the pages, I'd read aloud about Rose Red and Rose White, two sisters waiting for the prince and their future to arrive from *Grimm's Fairy Tales*; or, from *Greek Myths* about curious Pandora and the forbidden box; or, the *Bible Stories For Children* about Samson's strength and Delilah's betrayal. Grandmother fed me Oreo cookies, fantasy tales, and stubborn rebellion in her tower window.

I'd have thought mother would give up trying to change grandmother's ways, but no, Mom would say, "I can't let your grandmother eat herself to death." As if she had any control over what Grandmother or I ate. *Did I say, 'I'? I did, didn't I? I remember that I, too sneaked treats on my four mile walk home from the high school stopping for turtles at Pete's Candy Kitchen or elephant ears at the Fourth Street Bakery. I still sneak treats even though I know they are not good for me, but I was learning to eat apples now instead. Family patterns die hard.*

Would Grandmother be pleased that I'd become a social worker and not a journalist? I think not. She would have dismissed counseling with a wave of her regal hand because it was not a glamorous profession where one travels and sees the world.

I see interior worlds, Grandmother, and this fascinates me, I whisper in my journal. *But I must say, Grandmother, I'm enjoying pretending to be a photojournalist in Vegas this week seeing the sights.*

Grandmother always thought she knew what was worth saving and it wasn't people. She was quick to judge them as she had the McHugh's: "They never had any sense of what was worth saving." Instead, she sat hour after hour, day after day, creating beauty out of charred tables and remnants.

That's it! That's the truth about Grandmother that I missed as a child. My grandmother was a honest-to-goodness working artist. She was an artist whose quilts could have been hung on the walls of the Enigma, or even in an art museum with pride.

My grandmother, Amy G. Thuresson, would've been pleased that I finally understood that the second half of her life was not wasted spending her days in her second story window waving at passerby's like a Queen, all the while quilting, quilting. *How had I missed that truth of her life?*

As a child, I'd absorbed my mother's embarrassment of grandmother's obesity. Therefore, I had loved my grandmother, but I'd not honored her because I secretly knew that my mother was right. My grandmother was selfish to a fault, never dieted or exercised, and had no goals to improve herself or the community.

I had allowed Grandmother's weight and Mom's label of her being a prima donna to define her. I needed to reframe my view. Sitting in the Garden of the Enigma, I saw her humor, her ability to turn zucchini into bread, her friendships with her neighbors, her insistence about living in a castle with a view, her deep faith, and her love of fabric art. She'd known how to make her day into something, out of what my mother thought was nothing. Her life was filled with willful passions. It took real discipline and tons of stubbornness to live out her days on her own creative turf and terms.

Weighing lots was grandmother's genetic legacy, setting loose in my mother a fear of her and me becoming embarrassingly obese and immobile. I'm sure that's why Mom never let more than a pound or two creep on her small frame without immediately dieting and exercising, preferably swimming laps. She didn't understand why, when I became a mother that I ignored my extra pounds. But I did. *Was I repeating the female generational conflict? Was that conflict imbedded in me?*

But this did not mean neither Grandmother nor I lacked great discipline; she did when it came to her art and I did when it came to my life's work. I'd just never thought to separate her legacies before, just as I'd never thought about leaving my bed unmade, or that I'd become fat and diabetic by soothing myself with food in the Thuresson family tradition.

My journal was becoming white hot, burning up family fallacies. I vowed in writing that I'd take the best habits from both Mom and Grandmother and make peace between us. I'd continue to make my bed first thing, loving and honoring my mother who gave me the discipline of piano lessons, beds with hospital corners, and the joy of swimming laps. When I made my bed, I wouldn't only love, but honor my grandmother who transformed it into an *objet d'art*. Because I didn't want to become as huge as my grandmother, I'd diet and exercise as mom did. But Grandmother had opened yet another path for me to climb that I'd previously ignored, as surely as she'd ignored mother's fears. I'd become a fearless, second story woman. I'd find my voice sitting again in grandmother's side chair creating story quilts with color, pattern, and hymns of homecoming... "Abide with me, Fast falls the e-ven tide, The darkness deepens, Lord, with me abide! When other helpers fail and comforts flee, Help of the helpless oh, abide with me."

"One is not born a woman, one becomes one."
—Simone de Beauvoir

Chapter Five...Calling All Showgirls

I was becoming a member of the paparazzi tribe, clicking shutter after shutter of the natural beauties in the desert garden outside the Marjorie Barrick Museum of Natural History. I was particularly drawn to the honey locust with its rose-colored, fingernail-sized flowers growing in clusters. Besides admiring its looks, I even liked the sound of it on my tongue. Honey Locust.

Standing beside the honey locust was a mescal bean plant flowering in shades of lavender. The sign clearly said its hallucinogenic seeds were not to be picked. Wasn't that like waving a red flag at a bull? After all, this museum was on the campus of the University of Nevada Las Vegas (UNLV). However, there were other highs readily available on the Strip – free booze in the gaming rooms and expensive specialty highs. Perhaps the lowly mescal bean plant was safe in Marjorie's Garden.

Marjorie's Garden sported wooden bridges, jagged rocks, and free standing adobe walls that were constructed with irregular window openings of a cream and brick design. These stage props added shadow, depth, and playground equipment for its inhabitants. Sitting on a stone bench as a solitary audience of one, I delighted in the desert wrens' performances. They dipped in and out of the reflecting pools twirling, preening, and popping out of the window openings singing their version of "Oh What A Beautiful Morning." I couldn't have agreed more.

Here I was outside in February in my sandals, shorts, and sunglasses in a southwestern spotlight drinking in liquid warmth. Returning to Cleveland next week, I'd be well fortified with Vitamin D to withstand March's cold winter blast. I didn't even want to think about that it had snowed two more inches last night at home. Instead, I thought—*Wasn't*

I the clever one to have taken a winter vacation to these desert lands? That thought was followed by, *Don't get carried away on the congratulations, Carole.*

I sighed inwardly as I'd brought homework along today. I pulled out a book on building self-esteem in families by Jean Illsley Clarke. The night after I returned home from vacation, I was scheduled for a two hour training for the agency's foster parents.

This was typical behavior for me. *I may be on vacation but I always drag some work along. Talk about letting work define me. I just didn't know when to quit, did I?*

But, it's my turn to teach. I defended myself.

You could have traded times with the other trainer, Shelly.

But I hadn't, I sighed.

Get on with it, I reprimanded myself.

At least I'd started outlining a lesson plan on the plane. Clarke divided self-esteem into two parts: the BEING self (unconditional love) and the DOING self (confidence-building performance). In daily messages to children, Clarke contended that we often destroy self-esteem by marshmallowing (excusing our kids' behavior because they didn't or couldn't do it) or by criticizing (finding fault). This was in direct contrast to nurturing (offering belief that they will figure it out because they're capable of doing so) or structuring and protecting (giving educational directions to support expanding abilities).

As a parent I was good at the structuring and at giving choices messages. I was not good about saying next to nothing. I was a real chatterbox of knowing what was best. My children had often complained, "We heard it the first time, Mom."

Clarke went on to talk about shame. "Shame is a judgement about who we are, not about what we do." When filled with shame, as foster kids usually are, they learn to distrust love freely offered. (A common reaction to placement is feeling they must have done something terribly wrong.) Therefore, they feel they have to earn all love and be punished when they act up because they are never good enough for simple forgiveness or a second chance. They keep acting up until the caregiver can't stand it anymore and finally takes away a privilege, sending them to their room, or grounding them.

If the foster parent spanks them, they'll feel instant relief but foster parents are not allowed to hit for that very reason. Physical pain is not the answer to feeling better and doesn't nurture a child's ability to deal patiently with mistakes or misbehavior. Spanking, as placement often does, teaches fear and bullying behaviors as the facts of life.

This shame cycle needs to be broken, unhooking accomplishments as the only way to feel good about oneself. Children need to be loved so well, they'll learn to love themselves unconditionally.

Sounds simple, yet this is so hard. How to teach this to parents and children?

Then it hit me. It isn't a question of how to teach them. I need to teach this to myself because I am struggling with blame issues of my own.

I'd confided in a dear friend who said, "You sound as if you feel ashamed. Why? You didn't cause your diabetes."

Lamely, I shrugged and said, "I guess not." Then I changed the subject.

But deep inside, I knew that I was guilty. My sedentary ways and unlimited grazing had gotten me into big trouble. I was filled with self-recrimination.

Is that why I work so many hours, all the time? The more I work, the more distance I put from having to stop and acknowledge how I am feeling. On overdrive, I focus on doing good work and don't have much time to plan meals, let alone make the lasting changes that my body needs. Talk about a crisis in self-esteem. I don't love myself unconditionally. Self-love is all tangled up with weight and self-blame. I need to stop, listen, and change.

In Jean Clarke's categories, what messages was I giving myself?

What did you think would happen? You are carrying too much weight. I thought you had more self-discipline than to let yourself go to pot.

Criticism.

Read diabetic literature for understanding and new skills. Stick to healthy eating and an exercise program. Take time to heal.

Structuring & Protecting.

Poor me. Diabetes is a deadly disease that just runs in families. My obese grandmother probably had it. Tough break, kid. I'll probably eat myself to death, too.

Marshmallowing.

I will trust myself to know what I need. I will listen to my body. I am enough. I am.

Nurturing.

I wondered if our unconscious mind leads us to certain guides. This book was beyond a work assignment. This was what I longed to hear. In Vegas, I was eating right and swimming laps daily. I'd now practice *nurturing* affirmations.

I trust myself to know what I need.
I will listen to my body.
I am enough.

Clarke said the courage to talk about shame would free a person from its deadly venom. *Would I have the courage to come out of the closet about having diabetes? Would I share this example from my life with friends, co-workers, and foster parents?*

I picked up Clarke's book again, planning interactive parent/child lessons for the self-esteem workshop. When satisfied, I put the homework away and then bid the cheerful wrens goodbye to explore the museum before me.

'Oh, What A Beautiful Morning,' it was turning out to be.

In the entrance hallway leading to the main exhibits, a deadly sidewinder and a speckled rattlesnake were asleep in separate, glassed-in enclosures. Surrounded by the garden's desert beauty, one must never forget the deadly vipers that may come slithering at your feet not unlike marshmallowing and criticizing judgments. *Why did you let yourself go to pot? Am I eating myself to death?*

Unlike the live snakes, a stuffed horned owl sat in silent vigil in a landscaped unit. Raptors were in permanent flight in several others. An artist wearing a white T-shirt, chinos, and a red bandana headdress was camped out before an eagle careening down a canyon wall. Her pencil drawing captured the magnificent wing span.

"I can almost hear the eagle's call shrieking off your paper."

"An eagle never shrieks," she said not taking her eyes off her drawing.

"Yes, it does. At least that's how it sounds to me."

"An eagle has a limited voice range. It squawks. Auk. Auk." She shaded the wings.

"But, I've heard their eerie wail in the movies."

"Pure Hollywood. They substitute the haunting cry of the Red-tail Hawk for the eagle's guttural auk," she said giving me eye contact at last.

"No way." I stood in disbelief, yet knew this artist was speaking the truth. "They do a voice-over for the eagle?"

"Yep."

"Well, doesn't that beat all. When an eagle is not good enough as is, we all are in trouble."

"Nothing is really as it seems. My granddaddy taught me that a long time ago." She resumed drawing.

I wondered how else I was being duped and not just by Hollywood, but by myself. I was going to capture her granddaddy's belief and make it mine. *Nothing is as it seems. Like that little ice cream sundae treat wasn't really a treat at all. It was poison for a diabetic.*

In other museum rooms, traditional treasures of the Southwest were on display such as prehistoric Anasazi pottery, Navaho weavings, Paiute basketry, and Hopi Kachini dolls. I circled the art offerings of these ancient tribes admiring the varied designs and stories behind them printed on museum placards. They were representational gifts from artists who lived and claimed this desert territory, carving themselves into the lands' collective history.

I couldn't help but think that my Grandmother would have enjoyed this native folk art. I carefully photographed favorites to carry with me. After all, art appreciation was a new genetic legacy that I was claiming from my grandmother. I'd push beyond our sweet food rebellion learned in her castle window.

A new thought popped into my head. I smiled remembering that Mom had given me the same nurturing comment over and over again. I'd dismissed it not thinking it important or that it was a gift. When shopping in fabric stores, she'd always ask me to mix and match fabrics for her to sew, saying, "You have your grandmother's eye for color." *Thank you, Mom. I have an eye for color.*

Getting ready to leave, I noticed another exhibit room whose entrance was tucked into the left wing of the museum. A sign on an easel announced a temporary art exhibit entitled, *Showgirl.* A posted review by Draza Fratto O'Brien said, "The image evoked by the exhibition suggests though the idealized representations of women's bodies and faces are everywhere portrayed, outlined, or alluded to, woman herself is eclipsed by male fantasies." O'Brien went on to discuss that a typical female body is soft and round and this display was of "tall, sleek, angular bodies."

I always knew there was a reason that a Vegas Showgirl had never been on my job wish list. The exhibit displayed fifty-five artifacts of costumes, accessories, designer drawings, paintings, sculptures, and photographs. In all of the artifacts, long legs were a prerequisite. My *awk-awk*, short legs would not make the cut. No matter how much weight I lost, I'd never be able to sit, cross my legs at the knee, and freely swing one in an Audrey Hepburn pose. Nor could I wear a plumed headdress because even wearing a headband gave me a headache within a half-hour. Nor did my skin react well to lots of makeup. Instant zits.

Nor did I like to show off my curves, even when I had lovely curves. Nor did I sport long hair, preferring a cropped, tomboy look. Let's face it, I wasn't Vegas Showgirl material.

Instead, I looked like who I was, a social work administrator, solid in my white blouses and tailored business suits. In adulthood, I'd traded the buttoned down cardigans of my youth for business jackets worn over blouses buttoned almost to the chin. How sensible. How boring. How predictable. How sexless. *BINGO! Did I like looking weighty, a woman of substance? I wondered if I'd feel vulnerable if I lost all the excess weight?*

Recently, a makeover artist gave the female regulars on a Cleveland television talk show, a new look for the holidays. As I discussed parenting tips that aired every Friday, I was assigned to the makeover project. My brown hair was colored almost black. "We want to bring out your porcelain skin." Then he'd cut my hair into angles, shorter on one side than the other. The result reminded me of a Picasso drawing but I had to admit, it did slim my face. (I'd since let the cut grow out because it needed a weekly appointment to keep it shaped right. *Who had time for a weekly salon appointment?*)

The next stop on the holiday makeover tour was an exclusive dress shop that catered to small sizes.

"I want Carole in blue. We are looking for an Elizabeth Taylor look."

I sighed inside. Which phase of her life was I depicting? Not unlike me, Elizabeth came in many sizes. Blue after blue number was brought into the dressing room. None of them fit because the dresses were not big enough.

"Where's Carole? I want to see her in a low neckline, cocktail dress."

The salesgirl knew she had a challenge on her hands. I wondered if there'd be anything in this store that fit me. I grew nervous and tittered when she handed me a long black, not blue, skirt with an elastic waist. Finally, something that fit my no waistline figure. A glittery, black top floated over my long-waist torso. Voila! The deception worked. It slimmed my apple tummy, diabetic shape. The salesgirl added shiny jet and rhinestone earrings that dangled from my porcelain ear lobes. I felt chic. One moment later, I was crushed by the artist's reaction.

"I don't want Carole in black. Put her in blue."

The salesgirl came to my rescue. "We don't have a blue one, but doesn't she look smashing in this outfit?"

The day of the show, I was ordered to try on another blue number hand-picked by the makeover artist. It was skintight with lots of cleavage. I looked like a bad imitation of Dolly Parton with black Picasso hair.

"I can't wear this on the air," I said crossing my arms over my exposed chest. A distinct rip was heard as the zipper gave way. I thanked God for small miracles, as the black number was re-instated in the dressing room.

But even the black number proved treacherous. During my entrance from the backstage risers, I caught the high heel of a strappy shoe in the hem of the long skirt. I almost tumbled down three stair steps. Luckily, a backstage assistant held on to me, righted my footing, and unhooked the shoe from the hemline. Grateful that the skirt didn't slide off in a puddle at my feet, I made my grand entrance with a definite wobble. So much for grace and poise. A Vegas Showgirl, I was not.

I couldn't identify with the women in the exhibit who had chosen to wear tortuous shoes and fulfill male fantasies for a living. The black and white photo that was on the poster advertising the exhibit was of a showgirl and her four-year-old son. He'd been brought to mommy's work all dolled up in a suit, white shirt, and bow tie. *Her little man*, I thought. She had on an evening gown with a plunging neckline and a plumed helmet and their love for each other was evident in the eye lock caught by the photographer. As she joined the chorus line, she seemed to be saying, *I'll be right back*. Her son was adorable, but he looked out of place to me. *He belongs home in bed. Did this image represent for men, the mom they dreamed of having?*

I went on to an image of an aging showgirl applying make-up under harsh, dressing room lights. Tired smile lines and puffy eyes depicted a wilting beauty. Sadness rose up in me looking at this image of what once was. *How would I accept natural aging? Would I try to look what I no longer was? At least social workers didn't have to look young. In fact, some experience made us more believable, but that thought didn't make me feel better. I had always enjoyed feeling pretty as a young woman, and even as a woman of a certain weight. I certainly didn't want to feel all dried up and dismissed as an old prune-face.*

I wondered what retired showgirls did? Did they teach, hostess, wait tables? Did they quit if they found their own permanent Fred Astaire, Patrick Swayze, or John Travolta and went dancing every night? Did they go back to school and learn a new skill? Did they join the Red Hat Society movement and wear feathered boas and fancy hats still causing a stir when they entered the room? The red and purple chorus line of this 50-plus crowd refused to be ignored.

Then I spotted an art offering that became an instant favorite. Glassed in a shadow box frame, a pink feathered showgirl sparkled against a black velvet backdrop. Hanging from a satin rope, her purpose was to serve as a pretty air deodorizer swinging on a rearview mirror. This frame was labeled, "Beauty or Utility?"

This cracked me up. *What an ironic sense of humor. Beauty or Utility? Why couldn't it be both? Ms. Illsley Clarke said we needed both. Even June Cleaver did housework in her apron and pearls.* Well, if an answer needed to be chosen, beauty had won out in this instance because this pink showgirl was still in her plastic covering, unused, forever fresh. She was a real sleeping beauty who'd never been awakened to twirl and dance upon a rearview mirror. How off-putting was that? Lifeless, she was pinned like a dead butterfly against black velvet. *Male fantasies, indeed. The Stepford Wives revisited.*

Outside again in Marjorie's garden, I sat, opened my journal, and reflected about what I'd read, heard, and seen. I couldn't identify with the stiletto showgirl shoes and glamorous dresses. Why was that? Did I represent *utility woman*? Was I a female hypocrite who sat at a desk thinking work was more important than having fun? Why didn't I sit before a mirror with a makeup box in hand getting ready to dance my heart out? Had I become too comfortable in tailored clothes, sans makeup and Picasso haircuts that flattered my face?

Closing my journal, I heard the voices of the desert wrens again. Were their antics trying to tell me something? Were they calling all showgirls? Surely Vegas hosted line dancing at one of the many clubs. I'd ask the concierge and join the chorus line tonight.

On the way back to the hotel, I stopped at a nail salon and had the works. My finger and toenails glowed as rosy as the flowering honey locust. Once in my hotel room, I unpacked and pressed a cocktail dress that I'd last worn to a niece's wedding. While it wasn't blue, it did show off my curves. After all, I was in Vegas and as a member of the round and soft female tribe, I refused to be defined by a simple dichotomy of beauty or utility pinned against black velvet. Who wants to be one-dimensional? I yearned to be as multifaceted as a precious jewel. I would love myself tonight. *I am enough.*

"Be really whole
And all things will come to you."
—Lao-Tzu

Chapter Six...Finding My Colors

After a morning spent lolling in the Garden of the Enigma, I boarded a local bus with no particular destination in mind. I would see what I would see. Twenty minutes into this ride, a coed in blue jeans with a UNLV duffel bag of books departed at the corner of Flamingo and Maryland. I followed her lead, but I jogged off her path as she strode down Maryland.

This corner had tugged at me yesterday but I'd dismissed it because I was intent upon finding a nail salon. I'd wanted to explore it. Why? This corner seemed ordinary enough. Nothing unusual here: a florist shop, a palm reader, a bank, a travel agency, a coffeehouse, the "Buffalo Exchange," and a tanning salon. Tilting my face into the sun's natural heat lamp, I had to wonder who used a tanning salon in the middle of the desert. Maybe the ladies of the chorus worried about bikini lines needing a seamless tan for their costumes. Perhaps the night owls got up late and came in at 5:00 p.m. to obtain a healthy glow. Then again, "Why wouldn't there be a tanning salon in Vegas, the city of excesses?" Somehow it all made illogical sense in this city of make-believe.

For as long as I can remember I've liked visiting florist shops, so it became my first stop. The colors and earthy fragrances of flowering plants speak to an inner me. Posted on the wall in this shop was the Persian saying: "If you have two loaves of bread, sell one and buy a hyacinth."

Such extravagance, I thought. *But was it really? I think nothing of buying a box of pastry. Why not purchase a little beauty for pleasure?*

In a refrigerated floral case a single, white gardenia lay sheltered in a plastic box surrounded by vases of tall daisies, roses, and birds of paradise. It reminded me of prom and my first love. While other girls received carnations or roses that matched their dresses, I was fortunate to be introduced to the mystery of the gardenia that forever reminds me of youth and young love. *Wouldn't it be fun to liberate this gardenia in the large champagne glass in my hotel room? My room would smell heavenly and the fragrance would soak into my skin.*

Reluctantly, I bid goodbye to the gardenia. It'd be foolish to purchase it, as it would only wilt in this heat. I also decided to pass on the palm reader as I wasn't ready to hear someone's interpretation of my future, or perhaps I was a little superstitious. Instead, I opted to check out what was the "Buffalo Exchange" in my new calling as a photojournalist.

To my surprise, it was an upscale resale shop recycling designer and gently worn clothes. Since I avoid confrontations of being too big for my britches, I usually browse the accessory displays of jewelry, purses, and scarves in regular retail stores that don't carry grande sizes. After all, I didn't want to repeat the Elizabeth Taylor blue dress fiasco.

Wandering through the racks of well displayed merchandise, I found myself stopping and pulling some things that looked like they just might fit. Who knew, maybe something besides a long strand of beads would be possible? *And mom wasn't here to witness my comeuppance if nothing fit. I could hear her saying, "That's what happens when you let yourself go to pot."*

A half hour later, triumphant, I emerged from the dressing room wearing my finds, a pink shell top that was a light weight, cotton weave of double-meshed lace which slimmed me into pleasing curves and a pair of buttery soft jeans. I glowed, ecstatic with my size eighteen bottom and a shell top that wasn't a size 2X. Could it be that a slimmer me could now shop in regular retail stores? My body positively hummed with hosannas.

The clerk at the Buffalo Exchange was reading a well-worn copy of Joe Dominguey and Vicki Robin's, *Your Money Or Your Life.* Not familiar with the title, I asked her about it.

"This book has changed my life. You see I was trained as a beautician, but choose to work here where everyone participates in a profit sharing plan," she said bagging my clothes in recycled blue plastic. As I tucked them in my backpack, she told me more.

"I made more money as a beautician, but I spent more. I'd come home bone tired, feet hurting, and with a carryout dinner. Plus, I often snagged a magazine off the newsstand for a quick read before falling asleep." She tucked a strand of long hair behind her ear. "Now I go home, chop and stir-fry some vegetables with rice for dinner. And afterwards, I have enough energy to pursue my art as a weaver."

"And you learned this from reading this book?"

"Here," she said as she pulled from behind the counter another copy of *Your Money or Your Life*. "I pick up used copies to give away. Read, study, and use it."

"Let me pay you for it."

"No, please. I believe in sharing my good fortune every day. It always comes back twice fold."

"Really? Well, thank you. I'd like to be the cause of your good fortune today."

Accepting the gift, I knew where I was going next. Once settled in the coffeehouse, I scribbled in my journal, rejoicing about buying my first pair of jeans in twenty years. Sweatpants with an elastic waist were my casual attire. Perhaps diabetes wasn't the enemy. Perhaps this disease was a friendly foe forcing me into healthier habits and a good weight loss plan. *Thank you, diabetes, for getting me into blue jeans.* I couldn't believe I was thanking this traitor that had set up camp in my body.

Enjoying a coffee with steamed milk, I also couldn't believe that this new outfit had only cost me a total of ten dollars. I would have paid a $100 to feel and look this good. I could afford costly clothes again. But did I really want to spend money this way? This was a life priority question all right.

I randomly opened *Your Money or Your Life*. There on page 27 was a heading called, "Stations of the Crass." The "disease of materialism" was explained as looking for inner fulfillment in outer possessions. "It also comes from unconscious habit. Take gazingus pins. A gazingus pin is any item that you just can't pass by without buying." The authors said everyone has them. And you purchase them on every shopping outing and they all rest in a drawer, shelf, or closet along with your other gazingus pins. In my case, the gazingus pins were books, paper, pens, watches, and purses. I certainly didn't need all of them unless I was going to set up a stationery store some day. And the watches and purses? I was obsessed with time and earning a living. There never seemed to be enough of either time or money.

A friend had once said, "It's not how much you make, but are you able to live a desired lifestyle?" I had bought into this line of thinking complete with an expanding credit line, not unlike grazing into an expanding waistline. I never thought about reaching a crossover point to fiscal independence, saving more than I made to live off the interest some day. Who was kidding whom on a crossover point on a social worker's salary? Hey, an exhausted hairdresser had become a smart clerk and was doing it on a retail salary complete with a profit sharing plan. She made it seem possible.

Maybe, just maybe it was time to not only get myself into blue jeans, but also get myself into the green. Maybe then I really could become a freelance journalist and have enough green to get by. Our children had graduated from college and moved on. Life without children in residence could be a less expensive place to live. So far their absence was filling up with social events that used time and money indiscriminately, complete with a splurge vacation to Vegas. Maybe I needed to break out of my elementary "pink and blue" thinking and get into the green. I giggled. True to form I had purchased a pink top and blue jeans. Maybe they were my colors and not the beige that I'd become.

Pink and blue, after all, were my first colors. A substitute teacher whose name I couldn't begin to remember taught me my colors. I was in the third grade and it was Friday, the last class of the day at the end of a very long week without our beloved Miss Prell. The substitute passed out graph paper and asked us to choose two crayons.

Without hesitating, I chose pink and blue.

"Fill in the grids by alternating your two colors."

When finished, she put the grids around the room on the wooden lip of the chalkboards. Pink and blue, blue and pink, pink and blue repeated itself over and over again. I was amazed at how many people liked pink and blue. One person had used red and blue. A couple of the boys had used brown and black, which were ignored by the Sub as the self-appointed editor of good taste. I rather liked their solid look in a sea of pink and blue grids. Guess I still do, as those are the dominant colors of my wardrobe.

"There are so many color combinations to choose from but most of you chose the pedestrian pink and blue." Then the Sub picked up the solo yellow and green grid colored by Beverly Peterson, a shy girl whose deskwork had never been singled out before.

"Beverly chose differently. Bev is an original thinker and the colors go well together. Let's give Beverly a round of applause."

Beverly ducked her head while a lovely smile lit up her face.

Now granted, I was used to praise about my careful work and was instantly envious at the sound of the applause. But going beyond the Beverly envy, I heard what the Sub was saying even without knowing what "pedestrian" meant until I went home and looked it up in the dictionary.

Did I want to be a part of the elementary school crowd unable to choose beyond the "pedestrian" pinks and blues? Was I programmed to pick pink and blue? I wanted to be unique. I've never forgotten this lesson in thinking outside of the box, within the box, and beyond the usual. Thinking "pink and blue" jolts me awake when questioning whether a decision was really right for me. Albeit pedestrian, pink and blue are still my favorite colors. And, after all, my genetic legacy gave me an eye for color.

This day's primary colors in Vegas were not the typical turquoise, sand, coral, and silver of the desert. No, today's colors shouted blue, pink, and green to me. Wear blue jeans and land into the pink grid of good health and green grid of a bona fide savings plan.

Smiling, I closed my journal looking at the dominant colors of the coffee house which sported a huge, black and gold banner across its front window which read, "Grand Opening." The owner used the closing of my journal as a signal to approach my table. Introducing himself as Mr. Hogan, he offered me a cup of soup on the house.

"It's good," I said eating it slowly. "What do you call it?"

"It's V-6 Soup and the specialty of the house. You take the six freshest vegetables that you can find in the market and mix it with a tomato base."

"I think you have a winner."

I asked him about the grand opening and Hogan began telling me about his coffee shop, which was really the story of his career. Hogan had come to Vegas from the East to learn how to manage a grand hotel and land an overseas posting. He and his wife had family in Jersey, but she had agreed to this move because she felt the Vegas climate would alleviate her chronic asthma.

Hogan went on to describe the opportunities for hotel management students at the University of Nevada Las Vegas, which had a world class, hotel school that fed a booming industry.

"When I graduated, I was offered a London posting." He wiped at an imaginary spot on my table. "It wasn't to be."

"Why not? It was your dream job."

"My wife's health had improved and she wanted to stay here." He shrugged his shoulders and then looked me firmly in the eye. "She said that London would be damp and cold and that I'd never be home, anyway."

"You didn't go?"

"Oh, I went to London, but my wife stayed here and purchased a trailer for herself. She said when I was tired of globe trotting, she'd be here waiting. She found a part-time hostess job and took some art classes." He pointed to the entry wall across the room. "Those are her watercolors."

I didn't say anything. As a counselor, I do know when to be quiet. I continued sipping at the soup and waited for the rest of the story.

"I loved London, but the job was a thirty-hour day, seven days a week. Work became my life. I found out that London was cold and damp in more ways than one. So I quit the hotel business, returned to Vegas, drew up a business plan, and took out a loan to start this coffee house." He smiled at me and winked. "Coffee houses are the business of the next decade."

"No regrets?"

"It was a good decision. My wife's happy and I like being an owner where true quality control is possible."

"You don't miss the hotel business?" I had to ask.

"I miss the excitement, but not the daily hassles of running a big house."

Leaving, I thanked him for the unusually good soup and the coffee, adding, "You've achieved quality control in my book, both at work and at home." I lingered admiring his wife's watercolors and her courage. Settling herself in a trailer, she had landed herself in the pink grid of good health and the green grid of living within her means while honoring her spirit and creativity. I needed to learn how to find such simple peace by ignoring the beckoning spotlights of trying to do too much of everything. Perhaps that was another form of gazingus pins.

What happened to me in Vegas at the intersection of Flamingo and Maryland was a moment in synchronicity. As C. G. Jung defines it, synchronicity is "a meaningful coincidence of two or more events, when something other than the probability of chance is involved."

Instinctively, I'd been drawn to that corner and was relaxed enough to let the day just unfold before me. Seeing the palmist would have been as redundant as was a tanning salon in the desert because I learned not only about new futures, but gained the story seeds of how to get there. These seeds were now planted inside of me. Plus, the guidebook, *Your Money or Your Life*, was mine to use or discard. Which would it be?

Before going back to the hotel, I did make one more stop. I retraced my steps to the florist shop to rescue the gardenia. Somehow it had become imperative to release such fragrant beauty from its plastic shroud. My Vegas hotel room ended up smelling positively divine of first loves stirring within my soul.

"Books are more than books. They are the life, the very heart and core of ages past, the reason why men lived and worked and died, the essence and quintessence of their lives."
—Amy Lowell

Chapter Seven...A Must See Vegas Headliner

In my new role as a photojournalist, I was checking facts. For instance, what was the correct name of the mountains that I could see out the windows of my 23rd floor hotel room? Asking around, no one could agree on their identity. Needing answers to this and other questions, I began searching the yellow pages for a public library. Phoning the Clark County Library system, I learned there was a branch only a block east of the familiar Flamingo and Maryland intersection.

Headliner: *Vegas Tourist Visits Clark County Library.* I was probably the only traveler to Vegas that had put the library at the top of her must-see list, but I couldn't help myself. I find my soul stirred upon entering a library, not unlike others are stirred by entering an opera house, planetarium, greenhouse, theatre, art gallery, winery, or cathedral. I swoon over shelves of books soaring to the ceilings, the smell of the books themselves, the array of information accessed by touching the card catalogue computer, and pulling and tasting my selections for that hour, day, or week. So why wouldn't this tourist want to find the library?

When I reached the Clark County Library building, I began circling it in disbelief. This was a library? It looked like a museum paid from private rather than public funds. A reddish stone building with turquoise tiles surrounded by columns and covered walkways greeted visitors. One wing of this library contained the Jewel Box Theater seating 399 patrons in true theatre style. The Nevada Theater Arts troupe was staging a musical review, "Broadway Sings the Best of the Worst." This review was a compilation of hit songs that were part of Broadway flops, tunes such as "I'll Be Seeing You," "A Shine On Your Shoes," "More Than You Know," "April In Paris," and "Ten Cents A Dance." I liked the concept of hit songs coming out of plays that didn't make it. Even flops have unique strengths. Maybe this was one place where aging showgirls find a second life. That was another reason why I loved a library because it catered to no specific age; it was for everyone.

Walking around the building, I faced the parking lot and found the library's main entrance. *Leave it to Vegas to show off the backside first.* I entered and took the elevator to the children's floor where the best information is kept simple. A friendly children's librarian directed me to the history books on Vegas. Las Vegas is Spanish for "the meadows." Originally an oasis of natural meadows fed by a series of artesian wells, Native Americans, miners, and pioneers rested here. Beyond the meadows, was Death Valley on this desert's saucer-shaped Great Basin. Vegas seemed meant for dusty, beige me who had flopped gasping for breath onto the banks of my mid-life years.

The natural springs dried up in the seventies, not unlike the drying up of my pancreas production of insulin when it couldn't keep up with my overeating. Today's Vegas population, plus the over 28 million tourists, was supported by the diverted Colorado River water, provided by Hoover Dam. The mountains I could see from my twenty-third floor hotel window were the Spring Mountains. Well, back home, I'd been looking for spring, hadn't I? Vegas did have everything if I only ripped off my blinders.

Why didn't I play like this back home? Was there something more than diabetes wrong with me? I began singing the "no time" blues, but stopped myself mid-tune realizing that time was not the problem. I was the problem. Yesterday, I'd picked up two cards in the hotel's gift shop to put on my desk back home. One said, "There are a lot of things we don't have in life, but time is not one of them. Time is all we have," Jan Phillips. The other said, "Time is a friend, a healer, and maker of dreams," Flavia. I had time to play; I only needed to grab it, and make good times as I was doing in Vegas.

Taking the elevator downstairs, I went to the card catalogue computer, chastising myself. *Admit it, Carole. You are vain.* I wanted to see if my book on sibling rivalry resided in the Clark County Library of Las Vegas. Opening the authors' index, I typed my name in. It was here. I took down the numbers that were on its spine. Not finding it on the designated shelf, I discovered that I was checked out, still in circulation. "Not dead yet. Thank you very much," a saying from Carolyn See, one of my favorite authors popped into my head.

I collapsed in a vacant carrel, not realizing until I did so that I'd been barely breathing during this search. What if no one had checked me out for six or seven years? Would I be considered obsolete? As my breathing returned to normal, I traced the wooden surface before me with my fingers. I'd written my first parenting book in such a contraption in the Madison Branch Library back home. A carrel always focused and offered me a home plate to write upon without the everyday distractions that came with raising a family with a busy, color coordinated activity calendar. I had taken time for myself then.

I sat a while longer and thought about libraries and their meaning for me. Libraries had always been my haven. As a child, I'd read through the stacks in the Clinton Public Library although the head librarian there always fussed with my mother over my "adult" selections. I'd checked and rechecked out the novels of Pearl Buck.

"Leave her alone. She's read the whole children's section," touted my mom. "There's nothing wrong with letting Carole read the adult section. She wants to be a writer some day." My mother could be depended upon to be a lioness when overseeing her children's well-being.

So how come I wasn't writing anymore? My excuses to myself were that my full-time, social work career left me with little time for outside artistic pursuits. Working long hours, I had to be satisfied by being creative in developing programs, supervising staff, counseling, writing grants and preparing quarterly reports. But I'd written a book once upon a time and it was in this very library. When I'd been first published in my thirties, I told my husband, "I can die now. I have achieved my lifetime goal."

He looked at me, speechless. But holding that first book in my hands, I'd felt that way. I was an author whose book was in libraries that I didn't even know about; there was even one in Las Vegas. I glowed with an inner pride. I went on to write a Sunday column with my husband on adolescence for seven years in *The Plain Dealer*. I wrote a second book about the repetitive themes of a child's year to help parents better understand their children's behavior. Two months after *One Terrific Year* was released, my mom was diagnosed with ALS (Amyotrophic Lateral Sclerosis).

My life was turned upside down as my mom and dad moved to Cleveland to have family support during mom's last nine months of living. One brain cell after another extinguished itself, no longer stimulating the muscles in her throat and then her lungs. Without stimulation, her muscles shriveled up and died. Her ability to breathe became stagnant. The swimmer that she'd always been was drowning in a sea of carbon monoxide as she refused a respirator.

"What would be the purpose of getting hooked up to that?" she fixed the doctor with a stare, her mother look that broached no comment. "It won't bring my muscles back and I don't want to live that way."

In my Vegas carrel, I unzipped an inner compartment in my billfold and pulled out a published column that I'd written to honor my mother's many strengths.

A Mother's Presence

My teenage sons planted a dogwood tree outside my kitchen window five years ago on Mother's Day. Every year we would watch for it to bloom and it never did. Green leaves would appear, but no blossoms. We joked about our flowerless tree.

The dogwood flowered this year for the first time in pale creams and greens. It seemed fitting that the tree would choose to flower this Mother's Day. For this is the first Mother's Day that I don't have the comfort of my mother's presence, as she died last September. I can't pick up the phone and hear her voice. I can't send a box of her favorite chocolate-covered cherries with a card telling her on her day how much she means to me.

Shortly after her death, a friend gave me a sympathy card that read: "Separation: Your absence has gone through me, like thread through a needle. Everything I do is stitched with its color. (Merwin)"

That thought comforts me. My mother and I did say goodbye many times that last year, and in many ways.

Sitting by her hospital bed on the day before her death, tears ran down my face. I couldn't stop them. We were holding hands and she was staring at me with her blue eyes that always noticed everything, particularly anything that had to do with her children's well-being.

She haltingly said, "I can't cry with you. I don't have the strength."

A nurse came in. She put her arm on my shoulder and offered words of comfort. The nurse said something about being strong. I realized then that people other than my mother would now be encouraging me to be strong for whatever life would bring. I was losing my mother, but I would never forget those blue eyes stitching me forever into a loving mom stare.

A few years ago I was visiting an older son and went into the kitchen to get a glass of water. The glasses were in the first cupboard I opened next to the refrigerator. A wave of feeling overtook me. It was as if I had been in this kitchen before. In effect, I had. It was my kitchen, and it was my mom's kitchen. It wasn't just that this kitchen was equipped with my first set of dishes and crockpot that my mother had given me. My son had put things where mom and I kept them in our respective homes. *Glasses next to the refrigerator. Onions under the sink. Cooking oil, sugar and flour in the cupboard next to the stove. The kitchen was woven with traits of homecoming.*

My own home is interwoven with memories of mom's home. I have a chair my mother caned by following the directions out of a book from the library. As she stood soaking the strands of cane to soften them, as one would strands of spaghetti in a tub of water, I can still hear her words of advice, "If you can read, you can do anything."

I have what she called her discipline pillow on my couch. It is a pillow with an intricate, needlepoint design that she worked on whenever she felt the urge to smoke. She said it got her through the rough times of breaking a 20-year smoking habit. I have renamed that pillow. It is my inspiration pillow.

I also have my mother's first "Betty Crocker's Picture Cookbook." Its pages have yellowed and are smudged with big and little fingerprints. When I want to retreat to my childhood, I find the snickerdoodle cookie recipe or the recipe for a pot of vegetable soup. But, no matter how hard I try, I can't duplicate her lemon meringue pie.

Dad gave me Mom's cherished blue sapphire ring for Christmas saying she wanted me to have it. Its blue flash reminds me of her all-seeing eyes. Occasionally, I think it winks at me.

Looking at the shimmering dogwood tree, I bask in mom's announced presence. Today being Mother's Day, I will make a batch of snickerdoodles. Mom and cinnamon will find its way into every room. Mom has forever stitched our lives with blue ribbon memories."

Writing this essay helped me really feel my mom's presence in my life. I still grieve that she is gone, although I didn't miss her high expectations. I identify with Russell Baker who wrote: "My mother, dead now to this world but still roaming free in my mind, wakes me some mornings before daybreak. 'If there's one thing I can't stand, it's a quitter.' ... I feel the fury of her energy fighting the good-for-nothing idler within me who wants to go back to sleep...." I'd laughed reading this opening passage from *The Good Times* in my hotel bed yelling, *"How true! How true!"*

In the tradition of being a journalist in Vegas, I'd been reading Baker's account of being a newspaperman from 1947 to 1962 during America's "golden age of empire," the good times...provided you were white." I had read about his rise from paperboy to a columnist for *The New York Times* and in-between these assignments, his triumphant color commentator story of the coronation of Queen Elizabeth, whose name my mother gave me as a regal middle name. She had such hopes for her children. "If it's one thing I can't stand, it's a quitter."

The year that my mom died, so did the trade paperback company that was publishing my books. Winston Press of Minneapolis, a thriving publishing house with a strong backlist, was sold to HarperCollins of San Francisco to raise enough money to block a Ted Turner takeover of CBS; Winston Press was a subsidiary company of the network.

Bereft and overwhelmed by losses on both fronts, I literally threw my hands up in despair. *"I surrender."* My mom had no choice in the end as no one regains brain cells from ALS's steady progression of body atrophy. But I had a choice and I surrendered without even raising a white flag. I didn't fight back. I stopped lecturing, writing, and gave up my private counseling practice.

I took a salaried job in child welfare seeking order in the world where there was none. My world had spun out of my control. I abandoned the marketing of my second book, never visiting with the editors of HarperCollins of San Francisco. I no longer wrote early in the morning as the most satisfying way to start the day. Instead, I worked the mainstream hours of eight-to-six and lugged paperwork home and put in some more hours after dinner. I had become mom, organized and efficient, who always said she had no time to read a book. I had lost my childhood and become the next generation, all grown-up and serious. I no longer had the luxury of time to read, daydream, let alone write.

Thinking about these losses and what my life had become in a solitary library carrel in Vegas, I thought that maybe, just maybe, it was time to revive, to write another book. Why was I acting like a flop complete with a diagnosis of diabetes? *If there's one thing I can't stand, it's a quitter. I could hear Mom cheering me on as she and Russell Baker's mom joined forces.* There were still hit songs inside of me. I just needed to work at pulling them out. Big Daddy, my high school English teacher, had told me that if I became a social worker to support myself, I could still write.

"And when you are in your fifties, Carole, you'll have a mature voice with rich experiences." He'd straightened the books on his desk. "I write before and after work. You can, too."

Well, I was fifty now. There were hit songs inside of me that would give me hours of pleasure putting them down on paper. It took the Clark County Library to remind me of what has always been important to me.

I'd posted a saying from the Koran on my cluttered bulletin board at home. "A good word is like a good tree whose root is firmly fixed and whose top is in the sky." I needed to act on that advice and root myself again, to have a second, "coming-of-age" story. After all, "fifty is the youth of old age." I had lots of time left. Like that dogwood outside my kitchen window, I would bloom, again.

Headliner: Tourist Strikes Gold in Vegas Library.

Part Two

Second Helpings…Home Again in Cleveland

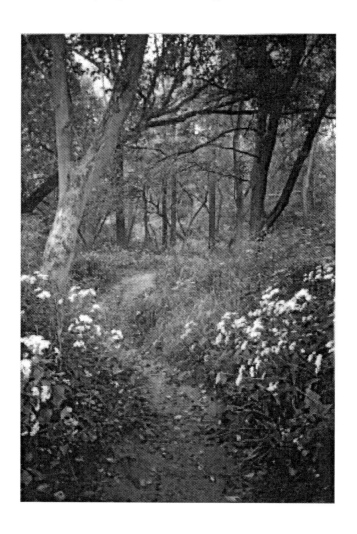

"What lies in our power to do, it lies in our power not to do."
—Aristotle

Chapter Eight...Vegas Curtain Call...Encore! Encore!

While sipping hot tea in a lovely Chinese restaurant on my last evening in Vegas, I'd opened my fortune cookie: "Your work interests can capture the highest status or prestige." My horoscope from the Las Vegas Review – Journal had read: "GEMINI (May 21—June 20): Write it! Let others know about your product, talent—if you don't blow your own horn, there won't be any music! New career opportunity revealed. Virgo plays an instrumental role." I'd stuck these messages in my journal. Good fortune awaited me.

Amused, I'd tried a few of the slot machines to cancel my need to return to my social work job. No dice. It had been a draw, winning some and losing some. I'd returned to my room satiated with having had a good vacation and feeling truly relaxed. What could have been better than this week off to play, read, and escape the winter blues in Vegas? And, my bonus had been the bliss I'd found in writing again.

Once home, Natalie Goldberg seemed to be speaking directly to me in the *Long Quiet Highway* when she wrote that Americans are fascinated by writers and writing, in part, due to their busyness. "Writing is a way to connect with our own minds, to discover what we really think, see, and feel, rather than what we think we *should* think, see, and feel. When we write we begin to taste the texture of our own mind. This can often be frightening."

I'd managed to slow myself down in Vegas, the city of twenty-four hour action with a colossal building boom created by tourism. As a tourist, I'd barely scraped its surface because I hadn't run around trying to cram it all in. I hadn't seen Ripley's Believe It or Not exhibit of over

4000 entries, the Liberace Museum, the tigers of Siegfried and Roy, the Folies Bergere, the Valley of Fire State Park to read ancient petroglyphs, or the Vegas Zoo. I had seen the neon cowboy sign that Lee Marvin shot full of holes with a bow and arrows from his hotel window, the marriage license bureau, the Garden of the Enigma, the Marjorie Barrick Natural History Museum with its Showgirl Exhibit, the Buffalo Exchange, and the Clark County Library. Yes, I came home full of the Vegas that I'd experienced with no regrets. In fact, I felt rejuvenated.

Was that because I'd written—processing experiences and good conversations in my Vegas journal, tasting the "texture of my own mind?" In so doing, had I de-stressed myself? New theories about stress are emerging. The old "flight/fight" theory was only one hypothesis. Researchers are finding that women handle stress in different ways such as "rest and digest." Dr. Jean Shinoda Bolen says, "While men may feel attacked, Women have a *tend and befriend* reaction—they want to talk about it and share ideas." Perhaps my stress had been so great that I'd used all the coping strategies:

1. I'm going anyway (fight).
2. Nothing could stop me; not even when I was reduced to going to Vegas all by myself (flight).
3. I moved at my pace and no one else's (rest).
4. I journaled every day (digest).
5. I examined my history, dreams, and place in the world (tend).
6. I reached out and listened to others, but most importantly reached out to my inner self (befriend).

Yet once home again and within the space of three months, I'd gotten firmly caught in the web of old habits by agreeing to chair another child welfare committee, eating lunch on the run, and rewarding myself for putting in long days with hot fudge sundaes with a maraschino cherry on top. I always, always found myself doing *just one more thing*. It's no wonder that my hemoglobin A1c had soared to a nine causing my internist to ask, "Whatever happened in Vegas? You're backsliding. I'm sending you to an endocrinologist."

Right after my vacation, I'd felt that I had to make up for lost time. Just looking at my desk piled with reports and memos produced a sinking sensation. *How long would it take me to catch up while doing the daily work, too?* Plus many of the staff had issues while I was gone and needed to see me as soon as possible to talk about possible child welfare interventions. I felt more than needed; I felt smothered. I felt on the constant verge of throwing up and wondered if it was worth it to go on vacation. Payback time was hell afterwards. I immersed myself once again in the paperwork and in supervision. And then I was asked by my peers to chair a child welfare research committee. Why had I agreed to do so?

I wasn't practicing any of the relaxing habits learned in Vegas and my body rebelled. I needed to remember how awful I was feeling right now because it wasn't unique to this particular day.

I consistently wiped myself out over and over again, as I couldn't seem to learn moderation. Last evening I'd been switching office furniture around to free up my larger office for two social workers and moving myself into a smaller office. We'd run out of room again and couldn't afford larger quarters. After finishing the moving tasks, I gathered the trash bags for one last trip to the dumpster out back. In bumbling through the back business equipment area, a long table used for sorting clipped my hip. *Ouch.* That did it! While I was in the moving mode, why not exchange it with a shorter table from the conference area? We needed the larger table there, anyway.

Just one more thing. As I lifted the table putting it on its side, a pain ran from my left heel up to my head, settling into the left side of my neck. It was still there whispering into my ear, *You had to do one thing more, didn't you? You couldn't wait until tomorrow when the staff could have helped you?*

This is a dysfunctional, all or nothing, habit. My husband pointed it out years ago.

"I hate doing errands with you. We finish the list and then you want to do just one more thing." He'd rolled his head and shoulders releasing tension. "You push me beyond my limit."

At the time, I resented this criticism, as there was always so much to do. I thought he just didn't get it. We stopped doing errands together. But I realize now that it was really me who didn't get it. My modus operandi was always being on the run. Get one more thing done. (My mom always said I'd learned to run instead of walking first.) My husband was right.

"You push me beyond my limit."

My neck responded—*Mine, too.*

It was about time that I understood in my bones—*I would never get everything done. There was always more to do.* That's why lists were invented. Stick to a manageable list and if something doesn't get done, put it on tomorrow's list.

Did I suffer from an attention deficit disorder? An anxiety disorder? It was probably a combination of the two with some perfectionist, compulsive disorder as an overlay. Regardless of the labels, what happens was, I'd wind myself up like a top and keep spinning until I was so dizzy that I'd go limp. I repeated this pattern over and over in over-working, over-doing, and over-committing myself. Then I reward myself with treats or an extra serving of food for energy because I needed a pick-me-up. This *just one more thing* habit made me a perfect candidate for diabetes.

My body compensated and then went into overdrive until my reserves were exhausted. According to diabetic literature, the onset of diabetes in type two patients was not that the pancreas didn't produce enough insulin; it had produced buckets of insulin trying to stay abreast of the quantity of food eaten until the pancreas finally went wacko. The pancreas had been dragged into the desert of over-eating and then abandoned. Exhausted, it had laid parched in the fiery fuel of too much food and body fat. While the pancreas croaked, the host body responded by becoming sluggish from the overdose of blood sugar. The feet became numb and were like bricks while the brain slowed to a crawl. Sitting and napping became the body's favorite recreational activities. Simple requests such as walking across parking lots and negotiating stair steps left the body panting, tongue swollen with thirst. The endocrine system was depleted. Literally, an *out to lunch* sign had been posted when a *gone fishing* sign was what was needed for my body to fast, rest, and recuperate.

Well, I'd rested in the Vegas meadows, but been increasingly on the run ever since. I needed to find a Garden of the Enigma to journal in at home. I needed to write because it felt good *to taste the texture of my mind.* I needed to change my ways and play well in Cleveland. I'd read once that new habits aren't about trying. One does not try to turn on a light. One either turns on the light or one doesn't. And I hadn't. *Turn the spotlights on, Carole. It's time for a Vegas encore.*

I sat in John's Diner, sipping coffee and massaging my sore neck, a new journal open before me. A handsome, young man with a mustache was drumming his fingers on the tabletop a booth over, driving me to distraction. (Maybe I should have gone to the library.) Dressed in a flannel shirt that still had its packaging creases, Mr. Handsome was joined by a man who reminded me of a coach with his crewcut and faded university sweatshirt. They exchanged greetings and talked boisterously about the Cleveland Browns. Then they got down to business. I was listening shamelessly because after all they'd destroyed my concentration.

The coach was a coach, but not the usual type. He was the young man's AA sponsor. They reviewed Handsome's past drinking and the young man's upcoming probation hearing. They discussed "the wife" and how he and she were getting along. She was giving him one more chance and was attending Al-Anon for support.

Handsome was on the mend, but had started to attend concerts and bars again. He swore that he hadn't been drinking, he just didn't want to miss the action.

"Stop right there."

"Why? I'm not doing anything wrong."

"Yes, you are," said the coach getting into Handsome's face. "You are just kidding yourself. Soon it will be just one beer, then two. You think you can control your drinking."

"I promise. I won't drink or smoke pot."

"You need to find new activities that aren't associated with your past binge episodes." The coach was definite. "No more bars and no more concerts. You need to work on the fourth step, take a moral and fearless inventory. Work on this inventory every night, right before the news, and going to bed sober."

Handsome started to protest.

"You need to feel what your drinking covers up. Being honest with yourself is the key to recovery."

The young man promised that he'd work the fourth step. Pencil slim, he sipped at his coffee and nibbled on some toast smothered in strawberry jam.

"You miss the excitement of your drinking."

Handsome's face lit up. He recalled past episodes of how it took ten people to put him down in a bar.

"See this scar? Let me tell you about the Rambo boyfriend of this beautiful girl that I went home with one night."

The coach listened, offering no opinion, nor judgment. Finally, he acknowledged the scar by saying, "You need to remember how you got that scar and how it could cost you your marriage."

"My Danielle is the best," Handsome smiled. "She has stuck by me despite my drinking. She knows I just need to be wild every once in awhile."

"Danielle needs you to be a man and get beyond being wild and all that means." The coach rolled his head and shoulders and said, "I believe that a man needs work, money, and a good woman. You have a good woman. You need to keep her and find the other two."

The young man lowered his voice to a whisper and leaned into the coach's space. I couldn't and shouldn't hear him. He was in confession now.

I tuned into myself and thought that Handsome was a ruin on the inside, not unlike myself. We just had different addictions. His was alcohol and other recreational drugs and mine was busyness and recreational eating. I couldn't have seconds of anything, any more than the young man could have one more beer without eventually creeping into a full-scale relapse. My addiction was adding layers of apple fat to my body that triggered diabetes. His addiction was creating excitement and intense mood swings. Mine quieted me for when the blood sugar soared, I slowed down to a crawl, often taking a nap.

The coach's firm voice broke into my thoughts. "Your past sponsors have said that you are very likeable, but you don't listen. How is it going to be this time?" he asked. "Are you going to work hard at staying sober?"

"I'm going to live right," said Handsome, "because then I'll land a good job and make me some real money."

"That's not automatic," said the coach. "You concentrate on building good habits and work skills to keep that good job when the higher power says the time is right."

Handsome sighed. "I've always been impatient."

"Get used to waiting," warned the coach. "The time table is out of your hands. Learn to work and wait, cherish your wife, and your life will become solid."

They left planning to go to an AA meeting the next evening, leaving me sitting in amazement. What were the odds that these two would be in John's Diner at the same time that I was? I needed to diet, exercise, and a take a fearless and moral inventory. They've given me a new mantra. *Diet, exercise, and journal fearlessly.*

Because if I was honest with myself, one of the reasons that Vegas was tripping me up was that I was sure I'd sell a travel article on Vegas. My fantasy of being a travel writer was on the rocks. A rejected manuscript was still making the rounds, and I'd felt crushed that it hadn't, and probably wasn't going to sell. The written rejections that I'd received said it was "too long," "does not meet our needs at this time."

Why did I think I could sell to a new market without credentials? Silly me. I'm like Handsome thinking if I show up, that's all there is to it. Selling free-lance writing is not that easy. And selling was not the real reason I wrote anyway.

I'd remember that I needed to write as much as I needed to breathe and not let rejections deter me. I needed to keep writing, if only for myself. Maybe then I'd find something worth sharing, something that was equivalent to "tend and befriend." And, I needed to pace my day and not always do one more thing. "Rest and digest" and forget the "fight/flight."

And while I was being honest, I also needed to face my fears of where all this introspection was leading me. Would I leave my job? I no longer wanted to work the on-call, long hours of child welfare. Was I using social work to hide out, where desperate needs always overwhelm me and make me feel I have no right to complain about unhappiness in my life?

Would I leave my husband who insists on being in his own bed at night and wouldn't travel with me? There was so much I wanted to see now that my thirst for travel had been awakened. Travel routes called to me, but not to him. Would this travel lust drive us apart? Did I want to travel solo?

After my trip to Vegas, I could go back to running around being busy doing endless work, or I could enter midlife in full-bloom in the PMZ zone of post-menopausal zest so labeled by Margaret Mead, one of my college heroines. Dr. Mary Pipher, pyschologist, cautioned that the surrounding culture might revere or burn at the stake the PMZ woman. "Many women regain their preadolescent authenticity with menopause. Because they are no longer beautiful objects occupied primarily with caring for others, they are free once again to become the subjects of their own lives."

Subject of my own life. Powerful words. I wanted to say "pretty" powerful words. Somehow the adjective "pretty" was still hanging out in my head. Was I afraid of becoming a graying, ponytail woman in running sneakers by age sixty? Would family and friends burn me at the stake? These anxiety-laden questions poured like a waterfall over my head. I couldn't let them scare me into being that which I no longer was. Instead, I'd use them to cleanse me of outdated ways of thinking and being and thus discover who I really was at fifty.

I dug urgently into my backpack and pulled out the packet of essays that spoke to me. To calm myself, I found the Andrew Wyeth interview published in *LIFE* magazine. Artist Andrew Wyeth traveled the same dozen miles painting new objects of interests as he re-looked and re-looked at his world. He never tired of his place in life and found much to his liking in his daily rounds. In his eightieth year of life, Andrew Wyeth talked with the reporter about how he now chose painting projects: The "flashes still happen as often as they use to. But I think. Wait a minute, does it fulfill the complete thing or is it just a moment of excitement? I weigh it for a while. As they say around here, don't take it abroad, just tow it."

I would learn to tow it. Take one step, change one outmoded habit at a time. I could *rest and digest*. I'd learn to stare at any false siren in my path and melt into a thicket of relaxation, content with just being here or anywhere else, at this time, in this place as I'd done in Vegas. Certainly, I could learn to embrace stillness protecting myself from a sore neck, a whacked-out pancreas, and a *just one more thing* syndrome. I'd slow down through journaling and its reflective perspective. I'd gift myself by living Aristotle's philosophy: "What lies in our power to do, it lies in our power not to do." I would develop the art of being still and fearlessly listen to my soul's directions. I'd enter the second half of my life through a second story window, a square journal of light, insight, and change. "Write it! Let others know about your product, talent."

Especially, let me know and help me develop the skills to do so.

I would be a second story woman being given a second chance, an encore, in the second half of life.

"Seek out... the inner voice which says, 'This is the real me,'
and when you have found that attitude, follow it."
—William James

Chapter Nine...Finding My Legs

I should have left work shortly after the phone tag calls with Mary Sue, my immediate boss. Talk about passive-aggressive behavior! Mary Sue could write the definitive textbook on it. It had taken me an hour to convince myself that I couldn't put off sharing my news until Monday because you never knew who'd get to her first. She diligently cultivated gossip with her peers at other agencies. I gave myself a pep talk and made the dreaded call. Of course, she wasn't available. Typical. I left what I hoped was a vague message about checking in before the weekend so she wouldn't get suspicious and phone around before she called.

That ploy seemed to work because she phoned me ten minutes later. I put my scripted notes before me. I knew her reaction wouldn't be positive no matter how I spun it. And it wasn't.

"I wish you'd consulted me first before turning down the nomination for presidency of the child welfare association."

"That's why I didn't." I paused, "I knew you'd talk me into accepting it."

There was silence on her end.

"Why didn't you take it?" She bore down on me. "We'd get the inside track from our largest referral county in the state. Why didn't you do this for the organization?"

I chose my words carefully, not wanting to get fired. "Bill, from the Phoenix Home, will be perfect in the role and he really wanted it. I made a powerful friend when I deferred to Bill." I paused, "Besides, I told you that I was elected to be on the six member executive committee. Plus, I'm chairing the research committee."

"Well, at least, there's that." She lapsed into silence.

I let her stew and said nothing. So far it was a draw.

"I guess I was wrong about you," she cackled over the wire. "I thought you were a leader, but you only want to be in on things, not take charge."

I wanted to jump through the phone and strangle her with the cord. After all, I was the only Regional Director who had grown a region so large that it had to be split in two. I gritted my teeth and kept still.

"Well, I'll tell the Director that you were elected to the executive committee," she paused for effect. "It'll be our secret that you turned down the presidency of the Cleveland Child Welfare Association."

Saying goodbye, I knew my next phone call needed to be to Ruth, the State Director and pronto.

She picked up right away. "Hi, Carole. It's always good to hear from you."

Getting right down to business, I said, "I turned down the nomination to be the president of the child welfare association, but managed to get myself re-elected to the executive committee."

"Of course they re-elected you," she said. "Besides, they know it's just a matter of time before you accept the presidency. Oh, here's Mary Sue coming through the door to share your good news with me."

I knew I'd done well on the damage control front and promised her we'd do lunch soon. However, I hadn't disagreed with Ruth about next time, even though I knew I didn't want the presidency. I didn't want to give 24/7 to the agency anymore, as Ruth did. I admired her capacity for working tirelessly on behalf of abused children. It was her life. It had been my life. But now I wanted a life outside of work. Would the emerging me be cut off at the knees? Perhaps the real question was, did I want to stay? Maybe Mary Sue was right about me after all. Maybe I didn't want to lead anymore.

I should have left work right after the phone calls and gone for a walk in the Metro Parks, but i hung around the edges of my office, mired in relief mixed with anxiety. Finally, I settled into the quarterly report that was due on Monday. I pushed on after everyone left because I didn't want to come back over the weekend to finish it up. I wanted it off my plate, ready for e-mailing on Monday morning. It was seven o'clock before I locked up.

Leaving the office late had been my pattern for the last three nights. Eating portion controlled breakfasts and lunches, I was arriving home starved. This late dinner routine caused my blood sugar to soar and get stuck in the high notes because I typically have seconds and then catnap in front of the television until bedtime. Because my husband had gone camping with one of our sons, I picked up a barbecued chicken, coleslaw, and ice cream on the way home. I grazed while watching an Arnold Schwarzenegger video where the good guy always wins. I kept stopping the video to go to the kitchen to get a little something more.

Once Arnold triumphed, the video channel switched automatically to the public television channel. By this time, I was limp, totally relaxed, and curled up in a red satin comforter in my recliner. When I woke up an hour later, a Cleveland Clinic panel on diabetes was in progress. How convenient. A guilt trip would surely follow. A doctor was discussing exercise and its value, especially since diabetics are at a high risk for heart attacks. He explained the mystery about blood sugar levels being elevated after walking. I thought that they were high because my body was burning fat converted to blood sugar. That had been a fantasy on my part. Silly me.

"Blood sugar levels go down immediately with exercise only if the patient achieves a consistent 'good'control range," said the doctor.

Obviously, I wasn't in the "good" range. My body was out of whack and didn't work efficiently. And it was certainly out of whack tonight. I didn't go for a walk, take a hot shower to wash away the stink of the day, or even sit down at the kitchen table to dine slowly to relieve my stress. Instead, I'd chosen a sedentary distraction and zoned out with food and Arnold in the recliner.

"Bodies just love exercise because it is a great stress reliever," said another white-coated doctor. "And stress raises blood sugar levels all on its own."

My ears pricked up. I hadn't known that stress in itself raises blood sugar levels.

"Epinephrine, a glucose-elevating hormone, is produced by the body when it feels under duress," said the second doctor. "This causes the body to demand more insulin to let more glucose into the cells for energy."

What was a body to do? I asked myself.

The doctor concluded, "Exercise, relaxation techniques, and eating sparingly help the patient during times of stress."

A member of the audience asked what type of exercise was recommended for diabetics.

"Biking and swimming are excellent choices," said the second doctor, "because they are non-weight bearing."

I started thinking about how I could handle my stress differently and my body's need for more exercise. I walked, but saw it as a chore.

It was just one more item added to my daily "must do" list. I loved swimming but hated dealing with wet, chlorinated hair. But, I did have a bike with flattened tires in the garage. And if I biked, I could exercise sitting down. That sounded more like it! A perfect, second story woman's exercise.

A dietitian preached: "Remember portions, portions, portions. Overeating is a problem because the diabetic can't handle an onslaught of food."

I glanced over at my ice cream dish. At least I hadn't eaten it directly out of the carton and some was still left in the freezer. But whom was I kidding? I had eaten gobs of yummy Fudge Ripple.

As photos of food portions were shown, the audience laughed. I laughed, too. But it really wasn't funny. This evening, I'd eaten enough for four people.

A third doctor was talking about the importance of wearing good shoes. I'd already decided that my doc had a foot obsession. Here was another endocrinologist talking about shoes. I perked right up when a member of the audience asked him to define "good shoes."

"Good shoes are shoes that support the feet. They are not high heels." He described a conversation with a diabetic lady and her insistence on high heels because she was only five foot one. She wanted more height. The doctor asked, "What will your height be with two amputated feet?"

The audience was silent except for a few nervous coughs. The laughter had disappeared.

Doctors specializing in diabetes continually warn of horrors that are commonplace in their specialty but not real to the newly diagnosed. The mind's resistance, or the failure to accommodate change, moved in. "Right. Like I'm really going to lose a foot." It was right up there with, "Who, me? Not a company woman?"

Clicking off the television, I poured myself a bubble bath. Undressing, I looked at my feet. My doc had recently examined my feet and fussed at me. "I told you not to wear heels."

How did she know that I was still wearing heels?
As if reading my mind, she'd said, "You have calluses on the balls of your feet."

"I've purchased and do wear tie shoes a lot now. " It was true that I'd recently purchased a new pair of black oxfords to wear with slacks. But, I wasn't wearing them with dresses because, *they looked ridiculous!*

Maybe I should stop wearing dresses. Now there's a thought worth considering.

She gave me some cream to work into the calluses on the balls of my feet and the dry skin on my heels. Unopened, I fished it out of the bathroom closet. I'd caress my feet into softness because I didn't have to suffer even though I'd turned down the presidency today and disappointed the boss, but not myself. (Rejoicing, I had protected my time. *I am enough.*)

Tomorrow was mine to play in Cleveland. I'd retrieve my bike and use my feet while I still had them. In the meantime, I creamed them until they tingled pleasantly. Then I tucked them safely under the covers, applauding myself for eating only half and not the whole pint of Fudge Ripple, and turning down a stressful assignment.

As I fell asleep I practiced saying, "No. No, Thank You. I can't take it on at this time." *Tow it for awhile, Carole. Tow it.*

Lounging in my robe the next morning, I fixed myself a leisurely breakfast and journaled about stress, good shoes, and biking. As a young woman, I'd biked all the time. But a husband and three kids later, I'd abandoned my bike to the garage clutter as surely as *The Velveteen Rabbit* in the Christmas stocking had been abandoned Christmas morning in the excitement of receiving fancier toys and family doings. Margary Williams's classic tale was about a rabbit that wanted to be cherished and find his legs. Instead, he had been discarded. But the bunny was rediscovered when the boy became sick and needed a comforting presence. *Well, guess who needed not a bunny but a bike again?*

After changing into sweats, I went into the garage and plucked my bike from behind the lawnmower, shovels, and rakes. I took some soft rags and a bucket of soapy water attacking the dingy blue and white frame until it was respectfully clean once more. After oiling the chain, I rolled it down the street to the gas station. Scott, the Manager, himself, came out from behind the counter.

"Let me fill those tires."

I felt like a decrepit, old lady being humored, but responded graciously.

"Thanks, Scott."

Then I pushed my bike to the bordering sidewalk and placed my wide bottom on the skinny bike seat. I wobbled off regaining confidence as the knack of bike riding came back to me as I rode around the neighborhood.

Feeling jaunty and my mind free of cobwebs, I returned home and retrieved my backpack from the attic. I loaded it with my journal, fine-line pens, a coin purse, lipstick, hairbrush, film, and my Vegas camera. Pleased with myself, I put my backpack into the bike basket and took off for the nearby entrance to the metroparks with beckoning bike trails. I passed by Stinchcomb Hill, former site of my daily walks. Gaining speed, I soared down Hogsback Lane into the valley below. The feel of the wind on my face hurling down the hill brought back the joy of bike riding. I was eleven-years-old again.

But the fifty-year-old me was puffing by the time I reached the next exit and walked my bike up out of the valley parkway. Digging my camera out of my backpack, I took a photo of the hill I'd just climbed documenting this beginning. Then I biked to a nearby coffee house collapsing in a chair by a sunny window after ordering iced, mint tea.

I pulled out my journal to write about biking and being eleven again. A motorcyclist parked his hog in a metered space. He removed his black helmet with silver thunderbolts painted on the sides and hooked it over his lambskin-covered seat. *(Wow! He knew comfort. I wondered where I could get one of those seats. My bottom was sore.)*

Dressed in jeans and a black leather jacket, he ambled into the coffeehouse and ordered a coffee latte. He, too, chose a window table. Pulling out a cellular phone, he proceeded to chat and laugh with a friend. He told stories while I wrote about our bikes. His blue and white Harley Davidson with black leather fringed handlebars and black leather saddlebags overshadowed and made puny, my Schwinn bike from the eighties. His bike boasted a speedometer and a clear plated, hooded windshield. As the Velveteen Rabbit had been made to feel "insignificant and commonplace," by the mechanical toys, so was I feeling insignificant and commonplace about my Shwinn bike. The biker and I were a study in contrasts. He was motorcyclist with power under his legs and I was a bicyclist looking for my legs. The Velveteen Rabbit had wanted legs because "The back of him was made all in one piece like a pincushion." I needed to get the rusty muscles in mine toned up for better use.

The motorcyclist drank his latte while I drank iced tea with "Sachmo blues" playing in the background. We were bikers, yet different. His rebellion, whether present in him or not, was there for the world to see, complete with tattoos curling out of his jacket sleeves onto his wrists, with a Harley Davidson parked outside, and with an ambling, attitude swagger. An efficient pancreas probably regulated his blood sugar levels. My poor pancreas could no longer compensate for my rebellious overeating that ultimately produced an apple-shaped me, my tattooed trademark.

As the doctor on television had said, the body had a serious problem when diabetes occurred. "There is no such thing as a touch of diabetes. There is no such thing as a borderline diabetic. There is no such thing as a little too much sugar." He compared diabetes with pregnancy. "One is or one is not pregnant."

I was a diabetic. The doctor had added that a diabetic needed intensive treatment at the onset. Diet changes, exercising, and drug therapy were needed. The last was the easiest to ask of the patient, as we are a culture where popping pills were the quick fix solution. This had certainly been my first solution but it wasn't working well, unless I dieted and exercised.

When I'd rewarded myself by going to Vegas to celebrate my renewed health and twenty-five pound weight loss, I hadn't realized then that I was onto something deeper. But now having written about my Vegas experience, I was no longer complacent, accepting my life as it was.

Last night, the doctor had preached, "Intensive Treatment was needed at the beginning of the diagnosis." He went on to say, "Every diabetic team needs a behaviorist to teach type 2 patients how to change behaviors."

I'd sat listening, not as a professional social worker and behaviorist by training, but as a diabetic patient. I was being a difficult patient in deep denial. I struggled with the shame of the diagnosis because I connected it with the sin of gluttony. *Oh, how I enjoyed food. Was that really so shameful? Was I really a glutton? Had I brought this disease on myself?*

Perhaps those questions could wait. What was important now was to accept my diagnosis and stop saying, "I'm just a borderline diabetic, a non-insulin diabetic."

Forget the qualifiers, disclaimers, Carole. You are diabetic.

Dieting was not new to me, nor was yo-yoing like I did after Vegas, because I'd never made "forever" lifestyle changes to keep the weight off. I remembered a saying from a lecture on resistance. "If at first you don't succeed, don't try, try again. Instead, try something else." I'd try something else. I'd learn from the Velveteen Rabbit about what it took to get *Real* and be a true companion to my body's recovery. When the boy was very sick with scarlet fever, the Velveteen Rabbit "knew that the Boy needed him...All sorts of delightful things he planned, and while the Boy lay half asleep he crept up close to the pillow and whispered them in his ear."

I'd whisper into paper and ride my "Old Faithful" bike. I'd exercise and write myself to health. Somehow, I'd eat less. My new behaviors would be a process for real and lasting body changes. I would make "forever" lifestyle habits integrating renewing behaviors into my daily routine. I vowed to exercise and write first thing in the morning like I had in Vegas, because I could think clearly with my mind uncluttered and spinning free during the first hours of a new day. An added benefit of this clear thinking time was that the day's priorities emerged creating a less stressful day.

I'd set my alarm, arising at five instead of six, and no longer would I arrive at work an hour early as was my practice. That would give me two hours to write and bike. I wouldn't get lulled into diabetic complacency with this new schedule of staying in touch with myself.

I was a social worker, a behaviorist, who knew all about measurable outcomes. I'd produce three pages of writing a day to discover what I really thought. I'd bike at least forty minutes a day. I'd watch my portions and not indulge in seconds.

Measurement of the success or failure of this plan would be told by my results in three months time. [1.] Improved lab glucose readings. [2.] Weight loss of the next ten pounds. [3.] Ninety pages of hand-written script to glean nuggets of insight. Why not use, rather than run away from my training as a social worker? My expertise would be my secret weapon.

Furthermore, I would be kind to myself remembering the Skin Horse's advice to the Velveteen Rabbit's question about getting to the state of being Real.

"Real isn't how you are made," said the Skin Horse. "It's a thing that happens to you. When a child loves you for a long, long time, not just to play with, but REALLY loves you, you become Real."

Getting *Real* and *finding my legs*, would be my pathway of accepting that I was diabetic and what needed to get done to get well. Plus, I'd love myself and expand who I was, now that I was no longer a full-time mother, full-time daughter, or full-time social worker. Now I could become a writer, biker, and maybe even a photographer. Who knew what might happen? The child that was within me, who'd become sedentary and serious, had been stuffed inside too long.

Loving that playful child would release her joy. I might even reward myself with a black leather jacket and black helmet with silver thunderbolts to officially declare my wild side for the entire world to see. I giggled. The biker looked over at me and smiled. *Being silly felt so good.*

*"My enthusiasms...constitute my reserves,
my unexploited resources, perhaps my future."*
—E .M. Cioran

Chapter Ten...Biking to the Borderline

The open window chilled my bedroom into a refrigerated icebox. The clock registered 6:00 a.m. After a solid two months of early morning bike riding, my body was screaming in protest. I felt like I was coming down with something ugly. My body cocooned itself in bed covers as I burrowed deeper, wanting more sleep. After all, it was Saturday and I could linger in bed. I could hear my husband puttering in the kitchen. If I was going to center myself in writing and bike riding before Saturday morning errands, I needed to get up. I repeated my mantras, "I am a writer," "My body loves movement," and "I will exercise both my mind and body."

I groaned and rolled over, tossing the covers off of me. Shivering, I pulled myself into a sitting position on the edge of my bed. I fought gravity chanting the phrase, "Resistance is the failure to accommodate change."

I didn't give in to my body's message. *Give me a break. Getting up at six on a Saturday isn't rational behavior. Whatever happened to the word, leisure, in your vocabulary and behavior?*

But I knew that going back to old behaviors was not sane. My blood sugar levels were now normal upon rising. My notebook was bulging with possible writing ideas. I'd be exhilarated in two hours if I followed my schedule rather than give in to another hour of sleep. I wanted to walk around the rest of the day, smug.

I pulled on a cozy sweat suit, laced up my tennis shoes, and grabbed my backpack. Yesterday, I'd spotted on my morning bike ride, a breakfast restaurant that opened at seven. Could it be my new Enigma? Could I write there, café-style just as Natalie Goldberg had in *Wild*

Mind? Inspiring thought. Maybe I'd just found the perfect behavioral reinforcer.

A grin surfaced from deep within. I was on to myself. I was rewarding myself with food. But if I was going to eat breakfast anyway, couldn't I go into a restaurant and order a sensible meal?

So there, Body. Let's get healthy and not worry about whether this is a crazy idea. We'll both enjoy a leisurely foray into cafe writing after a biking workout.

Rolling my bike outside into a traffic-free morning, I could hear the wind. The treetops were singing as they do in the Minnesota North Country, loud and clear. I didn't know they did that in Cleveland. Graying, mashed potato clouds covered the sky. Autumn leaves clung to the trees and ground in velvet clumps.

As I pushed off, I found myself shivering, but I'd soon be warm. I nodded at the occasional jogger and dog walker that I passed. Essentially though, the streets were mine. The noise of the trees hushed as I reached the valley floor after coasting down Hogsback Lane ready to pedal myself warm along the Valley Parkway trails. A lookout crow announced my presence in the clan's territory. "Intruder."

My bike tires were slick with moisture. The fallen leaves obliterated the bike trail boundaries. Shiny and wet, they were like snippets of wet satin ribbons to ride upon. My tires slid around so I slowed down, fearful of falling.

At the bridge, I dismounted and walked across, breathing deep cleansing breaths of the Valley Parkway. The river roared at me, foaming and churning in a Wagnerian chorus rush to Lake Erie. The river vaulted over its well-worn banks leaving still pools of ground water in its wake. The sky began to spit rain. I was out in the elements, instead of nestled in pillows. And I felt invigorated in a way that no amount of sleep would ever give me.

I pedaled cautiously on down the wooded trail. I struggled with the small inclines as my wheels didn't grip and my legs ached accompanied by shortness of breath. I focused on the thought of the cafe ahead. Fantasizing about becoming a regular, the server would know what and how I wanted my breakfast. I'd eat only what was on my plate and write without my usual distractions of throwing in a load of laundry or vacuuming the stairs. It'd be like having a mom again to ride there and know a chosen breakfast would be served hot with an ever-filled coffee cup. This "eating out" plan was a new diet connection for me. Maybe, just maybe, this routine would work. It would be like a turtle creeping across the land to cross the finish line.

Arriving at the restaurant aptly named, of all things, the *Borderline*, I howled with silent glee. No wonder this restaurant had been pulsating like a radar at me. It was fitting to eat here, ending my denial, once and for all, of being a *borderline* diabetic. Such sweet justice.

Entering, I matched the day because I was as soggy as the woods that I'd ridden through, but no one seemed to notice. I sat down, listening to the chatter and the turning of the newspaper pages of the early risers. I ordered two eggs scrambled, a single order of whole-wheat toast, and coffee. After the waitress left, a woman began to read an article aloud to her companion. She droned on and on.

A man at the next table stared at me to catch my attention. I nodded in agreement. He said to the woman, "Excuse me."

There was no response from the next table. I watched. What would happen next? Drama outside in the parkway, drama inside at the Borderline. *What a morning! And to think I almost stayed in bed.* He tried humor next. "Excuse me," he said loudly, refusing to be ignored. "I've already read that."

The woman looked at him and responded, "You could move." With that aside, she droned on with her reading. Her companion raised his paper masking his face.

The "Excuse Me" man was silent for another minute or two. I shrugged. What did I know as a newcomer here? He looked around and then began reading aloud the stock market numbers from his newspaper. When the woman stopped reading aloud, so did he. The server came by refilling everyone's coffee cups. The "Excuse Me" man ordered a muffin, re-claiming his table for at least another half-hour.

The Reader ignored him with her eyes. She talked at her companion, which was less annoying than the important cadence of her reading. I pulled out journal and pen to record what I had just witnessed. Natalie would have approved as she always encouraged writers to write about what you see and hear. Describe the table, the menu, the people. Just write. And so I did. I also wrote about how the Parkway was changing. Soon the crows would own the land and the trees would scrape like gray chalk against the winter sky.

While writing about the personal meaning of the Borderline, I delighted in the idea that coffee would be waiting as I came in out of the raw elements of the Parkway and that regulars would become like family, full of stories. I'd watch it all and record it as another season of my life unfolded before me, honoring therapist, Insoo Kim Berg's advice. "The illusion of choice in sidestepping resistance by making small changes makes it easier to do certain things."

After all, hadn't I discovered a fun destination that anchored the morning practices of biking and writing with a reward of breakfast? I, too, was a behaviorist who liked choices and could be flexible in my thinking, especially if eating at the Borderline was my reward. *This would certainly shush my body from complaining about the new, six a.m. routine.*

And despite my doctor's suggestion that I might find a better reward than eating out, I liked eating out. I'd start my day with a healthy breakfast that would meet everyone's approval—my doctor, my mother, and myself. I'd bike daily to the Borderline and get my diabetes under control through exercise, eating right, and writing myself home at the beginning of my day!

And what would happen when winter arrived? I would cross that hurdle later.

Right now, what was important was that I was managing my resistance and establishing new habits that practice would make perfect. It is often said that it takes three months to create a habit. Two down, and one to go. And, I'd found a Borderline destination guaranteeing the invention of a new me.

So I became a regular, easily sidestepping any resistance to my early morning exercise routine. When Kelly the waitress said, "I don't believe what I am seeing," I looked up from my journal.

There was Elvis dressed in a white suit trimmed with gold shoulder braid. His bell-bottoms flared from his accentuated waist and hips outlined in sequins. He'd strutted in for breakfast to meet a friend on Halloween Eve Day. His buddy, dressed in pin striped dress shirt and tie, hooted at his appearance. "You aren't going to work dressed like that?"

"Why not?" asked Elvis.

"You're crazy," his friend cautioned. "You'll get fired."

"No, I won't. I'm in sales, and the girls will love me. You'll see." He made a microphone fist and sang, "I ain't nothing but a hound dog, a crying all the time."

Kelly sidled over with coffee asking for an autograph. She had not dressed for Halloween, nor had I. But Elvis earned my respect for knowing how to embrace a seasonal celebration and have some fun, unafraid of looking out of the ordinary. Halloween was a good day to show some bravado and break all the rules.

I thought back to when I was seven, when breaking all the rules on Halloween had done me in. My body had hummed with excitement because not only was I going "Trick or Treating," I was going to a neighborhood party afterwards. Mom had made me an Indian dress with a fringed hem and sleeves on her Singer sewing machine. She had hand-sown beads into flowers and swirls onto the neckline. When I wore it, I would become Nokomis, Daughter of the Moon. I was in love with the sounds of the words of *Hiawatha* by Henry Wadsworth Longfellow. "By the shores of Gitche Gumee, By the shining Big-Sea Water, Stood the wigwam of Nokomis...." I'd pretend that I was Nokomis standing on the shores and bluffs of the M-i-s-s-i-s-s-i-p-p-i River in Clinton, Iowa while I recited *Hiawatha*. To complete my Native American appearance, my mom braided my hair with feathers.

Halloween was kids' night in my small town when instead of coming in when the streetlights went on, we were going out. Just thinking about it sent shiver fingers of excitement up and down my spine. And not only were we going out after dark, we were knocking on neighbors' doors and being given candy. All kinds of candy that was never seen at my house would be put into my open bag. Sno Caps, Lucky Lights, Milk Duds, Baby Ruth's, Snickers, Hershey Kisses, Red Hots, and Tootsie Pops would tumble into my possession. I could eat chocolate until my stomach swelled with contentment. Mom only kept licorice in the house for a candy treat and while I liked it, I liked chocolate better.

Mom gave us sloppy joe's and potato chips for a quick dinner. No vegetables, salad, or yucky green stuff. I was in eating heaven and all grin.

Dressed and ready to go as Nokomis, I repeated her words. "Ewa-yea! My little owlet!" I was going out into the dark to see..."the broad white road in heaven, Pathway of the ghosts, the shadows, Running straight across the heavens..."

Once outside, I forgot to look up, getting into the greedy spirit of the game of "Trick or Treat."

"We're never going to get to the party if you don't stop eating candy and begging to do one more block." My brother grew impatient with me. "Why do I have to have such a stubborn, little sister?"

We were one of the last to reach the party. Mom was there waiting for us ladling apple cider into paper cups.

"I don't want any," I told her.

"Nonsense. It's better for you than all that chocolate you've been eating."

After gulping it down, I ignored that my stomach felt funny and went to bob for apples. Cheeks flushed, I finally grabbed one with my teeth but got my braids and feathers soaked in the process. Mrs. Johnson gave me a towel and then pushed some hot chocolate on me. Well, she didn't have to push too hard. Miniature marshmallows floated on the top. I sipped it while waiting for my turn to play, "pin the tail on the black cat."

Blindfolded, I was spun around and the world went dizzy complete with flashing lights. I upchucked all my Halloween goodies. My mother was a seesaw of emotions and apologies to Mrs. Johnson as she mopped up her daughter's Halloween vomit from the rec room's linoleum floor. The party was over for me. My mother seemed embarrassed but pleased. She was pleased because I'd learned a lesson about what happens when you eat too many goodies. When I got home, I threw my Halloween loot into the garbage. Candy bars still call to me but I usually pass, not wanting to end up in another embarrassing moment. The smell of apple cider haunts me to this day, sending my stomach into automatic tailspins.

My beaded dress was ruined. Mom soaked and soaked the dress and finally used bleach on it. It came clean but it had lost its luster and had strange streaks of white. I'd disgraced myself and the legend of Nokomis, Daughter of the Moon by the age of seven.

But this Halloween, I was Nokomis already because I'd remembered to look up at the sky. Why Elvis didn't have anything on me for just yesterday I had a Nokomis experience. I hadn't thought of it in quite that way at the time. But it had been for I..."Heard the whispering of the pine-trees, Heard the lapping of the waters, Sounds of music, words of wonder; 'Minne-wawa!' said the pine-trees, 'Mudway-auhka!' said the water."

Yesterday, the wind greeted me as soon as I rolled my bike out of our attached garage depositing a leafy, slush pile at my feet and wheels. I laughed mounting my bike, helmet on, ready to ride with this challenging wind. At the top of Hogsback Lane, I abandoned myself to the hill, gripping the front bars but not the hand brakes. The wind hurled me down into the valley below as tears streamed from my eyes. I was eleven again and rode fearlessly. With no traffic sighted near the bottom, I swung wide onto the Valley Parkway and a half a mile down the road slipped into the bike trail as adeptly as any deer. I whistled, "Hello" to the crows and bid, "Good Morning" to the hardwood trees dressed and surrounded in autumn's splendor. The wind continued to play—lobbing leaves, sticks, and seedpods at me. Then the wind raced on ahead and had lain in wait to pounce on me again and again further up the trail. "Ewa-yea!"

With a heart beating wildly, I dismounted to slow myself down by taking my bike for a walk along an unknown foot trail. The wind doubled back not finished with me yet, pushing and tugging until it gave me a final push into a grove of golden yellow maple trees. I gasped. All around me, the sky was raining golden yellow, maple leaves.

Gently propping my bike against a tree trunk, I sat on a fallen log, mesmerized, an audience of one. I don't know how long I didn't move, but joy gurgled inside me at receiving this performance gift of the Parkway. The wind had playfully led me to an inner sanctum of beauty as close as a twenty-minute bike ride from my home. How many other moments of beauty was I ignoring?

The Parkway was teaching me to slow down, be still, observe nature, and breathe. It was teaching me that biking—not eating—was creating the energy that my body craved. How could I remember this lesson of finding a sanctuary of golden yellow tree light? It had filled me with a reign of autumn beauty. In my journal, I'd capture with words this performance piece of art to revisit this blessed sanctuary again and again. I pressed a golden leaf between the pages as a souvenir of this Parkway insight on nourishing my soul. Perhaps a breakfast out was just a destination and the true reward was getting there, being one with nature, and being Nokomis.

Last weekend, my husband raked oak and linden leaves all Sunday afternoon. He asked for my help, but I was glued to the living room couch. I was busy reading a book I wished I could have written by Ruth Reichl, *Tender To The Bone: Growing Up at the Table*. In this memoir, Ruth describes her need to learn how to cook, as her mother was the Queen of Mold. If I wrote a book about my growing up at the table would it be called, *Plump to the Bone*? I laughed out loud as Reichl's delicious sense of humor infected me.

No, I wasn't into leaf raking last Sunday, but I did feel guilty for not helping. I kept telling myself to keep my "day of rest" priorities straight, particularly because I was tired from a grueling workweek. And, raking leaves seemed too much of a chore. I knew I needed to refill my buckets by reading last Sunday, laughing and daydreaming. My husband said he understood but later in the week he complained to friends, "She sat like a Queen Bee with a box of bon-bons."

Actually, I was acting like a Queen, but I was munching on crunchy celery sticks while reading my eyes out. *But hey, if you can't take a kidding, you don't get to be Queen For A Day... tender at the bone.*

Viewing our lawn as I headed out this Halloween Eve Day, I'd laughed and saluted the wind that had gone elsewhere to play today.

Yesterday's autumn song had obliterated our clean lawn. It was a good choice to read last Sunday, storing good writing in my unconscious mind, because the lawn was again smothered in leaves. It would be my turn to rake this Sunday.

In processing "Queen For A Day" residual guilt with a girlfriend, as women are prone to do in the *tend and befriend* mode, my friend shared the following story. Her grandfather had raked and raked the yard of her childhood every fall. One year near the end of autumn, the leaves particularly troubled her grandfather. Frustrated that some leaves still clung to the front yard maple, he had gotten the ladder out of the garage, propped it against the trunk of this maple tree, and gathered the remaining leaves. When every leaf had been dutifully plucked, he climbed down and put the ladder back in its place. He then surveyed the clean yard, empty tree, and nodded in satisfaction. I'd had similar moments of this extreme, compulsive satisfaction myself—and it was always short-lived.

My friend felt sad. She was saddened by fall's clean up as if autumn had never been, and felt sadness for her grandfather who couldn't rest until everything was in its proper place while he waited for winter, snow shovel ready. There were no leaf piles for her to jump in as a child, just as there had been no chocolate bars in my mother's cupboards.

Yesterday's wild song of nature redistributed the leaves for enjoyment or displeasure. This metaphor of life told me I couldn't control the leaves, but I could control my reactions to fallen spirits and life's challenges. I was now ready to rake the yard to allow the grasses to renew themselves from deep inside the earth. Yards would always be there for me to work in and upon. Chocolate treats would always be around to take into my mouth if I wanted a taste of something sweet tomorrow, or the day after. I didn't need to gobble them all at once or rid myself of temptation by throwing my stash into the garbage. *All or nothing thinking is usually dangerous, but particularly so for me, a diabetic with a compromised food processing system.*

While raking this weekend, I'd remember that I was only here temporarily for my seasonal allotment. My husband could read a book this weekend or join with me in harvesting fall's colors. It wouldn't be a chore this weekend because I'd been to the forest and would remember the reign of golden leaves.

Maybe, just maybe, while raking this weekend, I'll make a bed of leaves for me to jump and dance in reciting *Hiawatha* into my pretend mic as I celebrate living well within my aging body.

"Ewa-yea! Minne-wawa!"

"Put your ear down close to your soul and listen hard."
—Anne Sexton

Chapter Eleven...The *Diet* Boss

Dieting did not come naturally to me. I fought food restrictions of any kind. After all, I was a grown-up now. As such, couldn't I eat what I wanted when I wanted? Apparently not! My blood sugars were still too high. I had the diabetic blues.

The endocrinologist doctor sent me to a dietician with my food diary.

"You're eating from all the healthy food groups and that's good." Then she paused, setting up laminated food samples on the table's surface, "My guess is that you're eating too much at any one time."

Gazing at the "Minnie Mouse" portions, I jested, "Why eat at all?"

"I know it's hard." She handed me a box. "That's why I'm giving you a scale to weigh your food."

Here I thought that I just needed to weigh myself. Silly me.

Together we discussed a diabetic exchange diet and portions, portions, portions. We also discussed several diet programs. She even recommended a few.

In the six weeks that followed, I ate more vegetables, weighed my food, and lost the regained twelve pounds. My body's metabolism then adjusted to the new regime, plateaued, and refused to shed anymore fat. *Typical! Now what?*

So, I joined a self-help group. Their diet regime was more restrictive, but hey, I already had the required scale. The next five pounds finally lost their grip and fell away.

The only flaw in the plan was that I now had a half a dozen new phone buddies. They called me instead of reaching for a candy bar, a bag of chips, or a pint of ice cream. They phoned when I wasn't even thinking of food and in turn triggered food desires.

Seven pounds heavier, I quit the group. The last thing I needed was more food prompts. Plus, I didn't like spending evenings on the phone because I got more than my fill of that at work. I craved solitude when not working.

Next, I tried a popular, weekly weigh-in program. The emphasis was on planning ahead. *Select your menu for a week. Make a grocery list. Stick to the plan.* I didn't last long on this one. *Where was spontaneity in eating? Wasn't this just too much work for something that was suppose to be one of life's pleasures?*

I did lose the seven pounds that I'd put on, but quit when I began yo-yoing, again rebelling against another diet's restrictive rules and making up new rules for myself. I was a diet dropout. Enter Roxanne.

Roxanne, a co-worker, lost twenty pounds following the Suzanne Somers's regime of selected food combinations.

"Forget about portions and just eat protein with veggies and fat, Carole."

Carbs were eaten with veggies only and fruits all by their lonesome self. This was a tempting diet because one could eat on this diet. A glimmer of hope lit up inside of me. *I could eat anywhere on this diet choosing what spoke to me at the time as long as I stuck to the proper food combinations. I could even have seconds.*

Inspired by Roxanne, several of us went on the Somers's diet. We established Friday Potluck Lunches eating only protein, veggies, and fat, sharing recipes and fun. I was in eating heaven again and my weight began to melt. I was on my way.

This diet was too good to be true. I added it to my morning practices of biking to the Borderline and journaling. I kept betting the staff that I'd grow Suzanne's long legs, too.

The greeting card came in the inter-office mail. After opening it, I was instantly uncomfortable. Under the "Happy Boss's Day" salutation was an earthen road winding through mauve and green fields against a warm blue sky. The card read:

> *This brings a wish for Boss's day*
> *And a special thank-you, too,*
> *For all the kind and supportive things*
> *You take the time to do.*

Because I didn't think of myself as a boss, the card jolted me. The national and state directors were the bosses, while I saw myself as a supervisor directing and cajoling first rate performances from the staff serving at-risk children and their families. I see the practice of social work as a craft, and at its best, an art form.

Why did this "boss" label make me uncomfortable? To me, boss meant dictatorial, domineering, overbearing, tyrannical, imperious, lordly, despotic, and pushy. I didn't like to see myself in those terms, even though I was indeed all of those things. Obviously, those descriptors were not the staff's intent. Instead they sent a card that pictured a journey along a road layered in kindness, beauty, and support. I paused and searched my memory banks. The nagging sliver of uneasiness about being a boss was real. Maybe this uneasiness was connected to dieting changes and the diet words of self control, will power, staying power, and wanting to be—yet not able—to be the boss of my menu choices. I wasn't sure I could change my eating forever even though I had to repair my health from adult-onset diabetes, the ultimate "hoof and mouth" disease. Overeating and couch potato behaviors had to go!

I'd recently received a workshop brochure that I'd tossed into the right hand, junk drawer of my desk instead of the wastebasket. I pulled it out. An addiction counselor was going to speak on the "Grandchildren of Alcoholics." His workshop would be on "control" issues in which blurred boundaries are a symptom. I was a grandchild of an alcoholic, paternal grandfather and a maternal grandmother who ate herself into a heart attack. Both my parents were the self-disciplined "heroes" of their families as the only children in their respective clans to go to college. Having met on the athletic fields of college, they went on to raise a "perfectly timed" family where order, routine, and control were big items on their agenda.

Control has always been an important theme of my family's heritage. I was weaned early at three months to drink from a cup that my mother held to my lips. And, I was bowel trained at six months. I always laughed when my mother offered this information because a child wasn't even physically ready to be trained at six months. It was she, rather than me, who was bowel-trained at six months.

Our family schedule went like this: Beds were always made first before breakfast. Breakfast was at seven, dinner at six, bedtime at nine, errands and hamburgers on Saturday, church every Sunday and a family fishing vacation in June. My days were predictable. My childhood was set and therefore looked safe. For the most part, it was safe. But the addiction counselor was right. When that schedule and its rules were not observed, boundaries blurred.

One such moment has played over and over again in my memory tapes. I suddenly knew why the word, "Boss," screamed from deep inside. I was four-years-old sitting on the top step of our local high school refusing to budge. (Parent educators often label this developmental stage as the Age of Bossism or First Adolescence.) I still had on my Sunday Best dress and patent leather shoes because I'd pleaded my case to wear them all day. It was Sunday, wasn't it?

My mom had caved in. "Just this once, you can wear it until suppertime." But she added, "No going outside and getting dirty."

Now, at the high school, we were in another test of wills. I was furious sitting at the top of the eighteen entrance steps, not believing that my mother had left me. Of course, I knew she would come back for me. After all, she was my mother.

It had all started over a maraschino cherry in the high school cafeteria. My mother needed to pull the hamburger out of the freezer and put it into the refrigerator to thaw overnight. Then it would be ready in the morning to make a thousand sloppy joe's for Monday's lunch. My brother and I had been dragged along with the promise of a maraschino cherry kept by the gallon in a glass jar in the walk-in, stainless steel refrigerator.

I took my time savoring the sweet orb in my mouth. When finished, I asked for seconds, please.

My mother said, "No seconds today. You barely ate your dinner."

We'd had a roasted leg of lamb and mint jelly for dinner. The smell of the lamb made me gag. I'd eaten as many bites as I was old by not breathing and swallowing them whole. And, the mint jelly was not strawberry jam, which I adored.

"But, I would like a second cherry, please."

"No. And that's final."

I turned sullen.

Finishing her task, my mother turned to leave. I balked.

"I want a second cherry." No please this time.

"Come along."

I followed at a funeral pace.

Outside at last, I sat down hard on the top cement step and refused to budge.

My mother said to move along.

I ignored her and my six-year-old brother who was now bug-eyed.

My mom and brother got into the car. My mother drove the car once around the circular driveway and then stopped again beneath the steps. I refused to look at them. Then mom drove off.

I sat frozen on the top step. I didn't cry. I didn't sing to keep myself company either. The only noise was the American flag snapping in the wind with the metal rings clicking against the flagpole. I felt as tossed about as that flag was, twisting and flapping in the wind. Had my mother truly left without me!

A strange car crawled around the circular driveway. I ignored the car and refused to respond to the greetings from the man inside. Unable to get a rise out of me, the driver took another look at me, and then left to park across the street. He got out, leaned against the rump of his car, lit a cigarette, and watched me.

Finally my mother returned. She rolled to a stop in front of the steps. I sat perfectly still on the top step in my Sunday Best. I looked straight through her watching the stranger flick his cigarette away, get back into his car, and pull away from the curb.

My mother had ascended the steps and was now staring down at me. My back stiffened with disdain. I didn't speak to her.

"Are you upset?"

I remained silent as a statue.

"You knew I would come back?"

To myself I thought, *Of course I did. You are my mother. But I can't believe that you ever left me in the first place. And if you only knew about the man parked across the street, you'd be upset.*

But I said nothing. "Get in the car."

Regally, I floated down the steps to the car. My brother didn't acknowledge my presence. He stared straight ahead. The fifteen-minute drive home took a long time. Once there, the household routine soothed Mom while I was sent to my room to change out of my Sunday Best and "think things over." I gladly went there, ramrod tall, and silent. Thoughts of a second maraschino cherry were long gone.

Something had shifted in me. That was the day I became the adult who would take care of myself. *I'd be my own boss. I'd go it alone and show her. I'd get my own jar of maraschino cherries and have one whenever I wanted one.*

Staring out the window at the maple tree, I knew that I was untouchable. I'd crossed over the line. My mom didn't have the power to control me. Like Grandmother Thuresson, I could treat myself.

That knowledge has been a big source of strength and a big source of weakness for me in the years that followed. I continued on that path, blocking fears, and becoming fiercely self-contained and independent. It propelled me to graduate school rather than a MRS. degree and into a traditional profession for women. I'd always be able to support myself rather than take a risk at being a completely dependent wife or a bohemian writer living on the edge of anywhere.

It weakened me because I never asked for second chances, even if I was on a wrong path. I'd blunder on and take my lumps, when refused another maraschino cherry. No wonder the connotation of "boss" for me was being bossy beyond belief! It certainly didn't make me feel loveable.

The staff greeting card offered a different view of being a "boss." Could I be kind and supportive to myself in learning how to eat and think differently about dieting? Rigid controls. Blurring boundaries. I had it all wrong. The girl left sitting on the cold stone steps was not scoffing at her mom acting righteous, but was really afraid. She was so vulnerable sitting there alone, wary of the stranger. She bear-hugged herself into staying in control. If she'd cried, her mother would have taken control, held, and soothed her.

But by not crying or even speaking, that little girl made her mother angrier, and so became a bossy four-year-old, forever sitting still on cold, hard steps. Banished to her room hardened her resolve. And so, the life stage had been set and the choice was always the same. Dependence was not to be born. Clinging behavior was not my style.

Eventually I can to see that my use of all-or-nothing thinking needed to be shattered. If I goofed on my way to exercising and eating right, I needed to be kind to myself. I'd forgive myself, pick myself up, and not let the prima donna inside scold me into sitting on stone cold steps, forever a bratty, unlovable girl.

Was I strong enough to diet? This was the wrong question. I had more than enough self-restraint. I needed to remember the little girl, who sat with courage beyond her years, sitting frozen and abandoned. I'd honor and thaw that brazen girl within me.

Yes, the greeting card from the staff was right on target. *It was a Happy Boss's Day!* Maybe I'd grow up at last. Then I could choose what kind of boss I wanted to be to myself. I'd take that little girl's hand and lead her down the steps knowing that having a second maraschino cherry was not possible. And though not possible, it wouldn't be the end of the world she wanted.

I'd remember that life had more than one kind of maraschino cherry. Life gave second chances, even if not second helpings, to an adult diabetic who needed to become a kind and supportive boss of herself on the path to getting well. Perhaps I could get it right this time by being a bratty, good girl staring down the diabetic stranger within myself.

So, Suzanne Somers, if I eat a carb with a protein, I won't chastise myself. I'll just get on with your combination diet plan. And if I choose another diet plan, I won't balk at the rules, portion sizes, or menu planning. I won't stiffen, argue, and blur the boundaries getting nowhere but left behind, gaining weight, and no wisdom. I'd remember what the real question was. It was not—Could I stay on a diet? It was—Did I want to pay the consequences of not dieting?

"Belief conditions experience, and experience then strengthens belief. What you believe, you experience."
—Krishnamurti

Chapter Twelve...The Volatiles of Life

I lost weight on the Suzanne Somers's diet. My daily blood sugar readings were dramatically lower. Flushed with success, I continued to eat differently than my friends and family. But I'd be lying if I said I didn't miss a turkey club, double-decker sandwich with chips, or a baked potato swimming in butter and sour cream, or spaghetti with spicy meatballs. I feared it was only a matter of time before I rebelled and reverted to eating familiar, satisfying food combinations. As further proof that this dieting experiment was overwhelming me, I'd begun reading cookbooks as a leisure activity, and so my sleep was flooded with food dreams. These were not good signs.

One dream disturbed me with regularity. I was at a picnic in the backyard of my childhood. Mom, my brother, and Jens Juhl watched me. Why were they staring? Although troubled by this repetitive dream, I dismissed it because my food selections were drawing enough uncomfortable stares and comments in real life.

"Bring Carole a fork," the hostess would say. "She's not having a bun with her hamburger."

Waving the fork off, I wrapped the hamburger in lettuce.

"But I purchased a sugarless pie just for you because I knew you were on a diet," said a dear friend.

"How sweet of you. But, I can't eat one more bite of anything." *I rubbed my belly to emphasize my words hoping I really was stuffed and wouldn't go home and binge on popcorn. But if I did, it was only popcorn. Better for me than pie, wasn't it?*

"You don't know what you're missing," said my husband. "This pizza is delicious."

"It looks like it is, but I can't get enough of this tasty salad." *I hoped I wouldn't be struck dead for lying.*

Sometimes, I apologized to the hostess saying that my stomach was touchy, but nothing contagious. Just a reaction to a new medication. Sometimes, I suggested to friends that we eat out, which avoided home dinner gatherings and inflexible menus altogether. Sometimes I just became angry and said my doctor put me on a restrictive diet and not to worry about me. And, sometimes, when all else failed, I announced, "I'm a diabetic. Please don't push food at me that I can't have."

That always silenced the room. I felt contrite later wondering if I'd ever be invited anywhere again. *Anger was reducing me to that bossy, four-year-old sitting on the steps to nowhere warm and inviting. I hated having the food on my plate questioned as a topic of discussion. It wasn't my stomach that was touchy. Instead, it was me, all me.*

No wonder I was having food dreams. No wonder I was worried about this food combination regime that was working for me. It was just a matter of time before the Somers' diet would be tossed in the garbage along with the sugarless pie sent home to eat when I wasn't so full. This combination diet was a hassle and I hated food hassles. This diet was causing me problems and I didn't really want to be a Vegas showgirl. Or did I?

I began collecting advice from the skinny people for new ways of thinking and behaving. My forever thin, former college roommate said she always left half of what she was served on her plate. "Or, I order one meal and talk my husband into splitting it with me."

"Patti eats like a bird," boasted her husband.

I don't think anyone has ever said that about me.

Another thin friend, Marilyn, said, "I always re-arrange my food. I never eat what I don't want and no one notices because it looks like I'm eating everything, then get full, and can't eat any more." She demonstrated by cutting up her asparagus into a dozen bites and pushed it around, never taking a bite of it.

It was an amazing demonstration. Now you see it, now you don't. You think she ate it.

"The hostess never gets offended because I've enjoyed my meal. What I don't eat, I use to decorate my plate, with no one the wiser."

Could I do that? I'd have to give up my life-long membership to Mom's Clean Plate Club. I came from a long line of women who prided themselves on preparing irresistible meals. You'd think that the meal presented determined their worth! Now that I thought about this connection, I know that they did think that! Did I think that too?

A television celebrity said he always ate for an hour of something healthy like an apple, a banana, or steamed vegetables an hour before going to a party. Full, he ignored the food around him. Instead, he worked the room and talked to everyone.

Me? Go to a party and not eat? Doesn't a party mean fun food? Isn't a party for eating and laughing together? Could it be that I could concentrate on the socializing, and not what's on my plate?

Portion control. Healthy food choices. Suzanne Somers's combination diet or not, I was shrinking my stomach. I welcomed my stomach feeling taut like a drum skin shrinking and radiating a persistent dull thud of discomfort. My appetite, fearing extinction, would echo my stomach's distress sending short spurts of anxiety from deep within. This was my appetite calling, not true hunger. I'd ignore this call and find something better to do than to eat. Determined, I'd push away from the table to bike, shoot photos, or take a bubble bath. The behaviorist in me had a list of better things to do to satisfy me.

Then came the day I found myself eating brussels sprout's on automatic pilot. I was reading a good book and swallowed those suckers almost whole. I hated brussels sprout's despite all the good nutrients they offered. Getting out my journal, I began scribbling about how I often ate without really tasting my food. Brussels sprouts were one thing, but I also did this swallowing act with popcorn, which I adored. I often crammed fistfuls of it into my mouth as if I couldn't get enough.

Maybe I over-ate because I didn't recognize when I was full because I was often doing two things at a time, such as eating while reading. Eating while doing paperwork. Eating while watching television. Eating while talking on the phone. Eating became the secondary rather than the primary activity. Maybe I needed to rethink this habit of inhaling food.

"Slow down and enjoy your food," the dietician had said. "Chew each bite twenty times."

"Twenty times?" I asked. She couldn't mean it.

"Well, maybe not twenty, but how about at least ten?"

She said research showed that chewing a lot and taking a deep whiff of your food pushed aromatic molecules, called the volatiles, up into your nose.

"The olfactory bulb behind the bridge of the nose is where a lot of flavor perception takes place."

As a child, I must have shut this bulb down not wanting to taste chalk when drinking milk or taste the yucky gristle of egg whites. I'd learned as a child to eat without tasting by swallowing bites of food whole as I'd been doing with the brussels sprouts.

Bingo. The annual spring picnic of my childhood unfolded in my mind. I now knew why the staring dream was haunting me and it had nothing and everything to do with the Suzanne Somers' diet. Eating differently always meant trouble for me.

When I was eight, I had a thing about milk. I hated the taste of it, but could tolerate "Borden's." The one where, Elsie, the daisy-crowned cow was featured on the front of the carton. This brand preference irritated my mother because they didn't carry "Borden's" at her favorite supermarket and she complained that she had to make a special stop for it. My grandmother had turned me onto "Borden's" when I visited at her apartment. As a youngster, I was a finicky eater and refused milk if it wasn't "Borden's."

"Milk is milk and there is no difference between brands," argued Mom.

" I can taste the difference," I retorted. The others turned chalky in my mouth and left a bad aftertaste. I wanted to spit it out, but I knew that would cause big trouble with Mom. I just refused to drink what I, as an eight-year-old connoisseur of milk, considered an off-brand. Actually, I would have preferred to refuse all milk. Or, if I had to drink it, I liked Oreo cookies with it. But I was told that would ruin my appetite for dinner. Besides Mom seldom permitted "Oreos" in the house.

My mother and I certainly had a history of getting "stubborn" about food. I remember having to sit with a sunnyside up egg in front of me for breakfast because I wasn't allowed to leave the table until I cleaned my plate. There was no offending milk before me because any kind of milk at breakfast was enough to produce vomiting reflexes.

I didn't particularly like eggs, either, so I would sit with the yolk staring at me and me staring at it while I nibbled at toast. I was labeled as "being difficult." The longer I sat, the colder the egg got. The yolk congealed and was better cold, but the white field surrounding it turned to slippery ice. I knew my mom would win as my friends, JeriKay and Linda, would be arriving soon and I didn't want to miss walking to school with them.

I closed my eyes and held my nose. *(I must have instinctively known about volatiles getting up my nose at age eight.)* I stuffed the graying gristle down trying not to think about what I was eating. Hurriedly I excused myself to brush my teeth gagging at the bathroom sink. Nothing came up. It stayed in my throat the rest of the morning, every morning.

My father finally came to my rescue and suggested that I eat my breakfast egg hot by slipping my toast under it; its taste diluted by the toast. Finished with the nasty egg, I asked, and reluctantly received a second piece of toast with jam as an enjoyable breakfast reward.

Mom reminded me that two pieces of toast wasn't a good habit to get into. "Lots of calories there."

"But I'm skinny."

"For now," Mom made sure she had the last word. A few months later, mom stopped serving me a sunnyside up egg. We reached a breakfast accord. She began giving me homemade vegetable soup for breakfast with one slice of toast.

"Thanks, Mom, I love soup." The breakfast table became peaceful.

In the meantime, I continued to struggle with milk and its chalky taste.

Every May when the rhubarb came up in the side yard of my childhood home, our next door neighbor, Jens Juhl, cut the first pink stalks with his pen knife and took them to my mother. A master baker, mother's task was to produce a pie with the rhubarb bubbling up and peeking through the lattice pastry top.

Jens scrubbed the picnic table and I set it in eager anticipation of this annual rite of spring. Mom and Marie Juhl placed a picnic feast under the budding maple tree. We had potato salad, celery seed coleslaw, watermelon pickles, baked beans, sunshine Jell-O and grilled hamburgers. Jens and I were enjoying everything, but saved room for dessert. My brother John asked if I wanted some milk. I said, "Not now. I'll have some later with my pie."

I thought it was strange that he was pushing milk at me, but who cared? He wasn't going to trigger a scene today from me. Winter was over. The baby green leaves of my climbing maple tree would soon provide a backyard refuge. My bike and roller skates were reactivated for the season. I was home free. No more leggings, wool mittens, and heavy boots to weigh me down.

My mother cut the pie, and spring officially filled the air. Jens winked at me as Mom placed warm slices in front of us. She poured me a glass of milk from the "Borden's" container with Elsie smiling at me under her crown of daisies. I smiled back while gulping a swallow of milk concentrating on my pie. The milk tasted like chalk. I wondered if it had gotten too warm setting on the picnic table, but I shrugged it off thinking, who cared when the taste of spring was before me?

Maybe I could even get away with spilling some of it on the grass when no one was looking.

My pesky brother asked, "How is it?"

"Wonderful." I smiled at Jens and turned to my mom; "This pie is the best ever."

"How's your milk?" she asked.

"Fine. Fine," I lied. "Thanks for getting 'Borden's.' You know how I hate the other stuff."

"It is the other stuff!" my brother shrieked. "I knew she couldn't tell the difference." My brother and my mom had put different milk in the "Borden's" container.

Mom and I never discussed milk again, and "Borden's" was forever banished from our home. She bought her preferred milk only. (As an adult, I now know that she'd effectively eliminated cream from my diet because her preferred brand had a lower fat count. That's why it tasted like chalk.) But at age eight, I learned to swallow Mom's blue milk and to eat what was put before me. Winter had returned without my ever knowing it at the table of my childhood. I ate what was set before me and swallowed any struggle with food. I gave up creating food scenes and being a finicky eater. I ate indiscriminately, distracting myself by talking with my dad, making up stories in my head, or reading a book at the table if I could get away with it, not tasting the food I disliked.

In *Feeding the Hungry Heart*, author Geneen Roth, who must have sat at my childhood table with me, wrote that, "The drive to eat compulsively is not an uncontrollable instinct; it is a cry for help...You've got to feel that you're worth your own time...Are your needs just as important as your mother's?...Or are you going to continue smothering yourself with food?...Do you have to die to get what you want?"

I was smothering myself with food. Mom had effectively passed on her belief that I'd recklessly become as fat as my grandmother had if I didn't watch out. I'd taken on her daily struggles with food as my struggle, constantly yearning for treats and vowing to never go on Mom's constant diets of eggs and spinach, 800 calories or less, etc.

Would I ever be slim again? I didn't want to kill myself piece-by-piece. I wanted to become a finicky eater without causing moms and friends trouble at the table. Then again, why shouldn't a loved one fuss and make me what I liked? Or why couldn't I become guilt-free like Marilyn and decorate my plate with uneaten food? I wanted to stop feeling guilty about whatever I put in my mouth.

I needed to work on taking ownership of where my food capitulation had led me and put an end to it because I was hurting my body, my life, and myself. I may have won the food battle with my mom by eating on automatic pilot, but I'd certainly lost the war. And Mom was gone now.

Was I holding onto the struggle to keep her alive within me? Ouch! That's a heavy thought. Could it be a true? I hoped not. I only knew for sure that Krishnamurti was right when he said, "Belief conditions experience and experience then strengthens belief. What you believe, you experience."

Another thing that I knew for sure was—being big was no longer beautiful and luxurious for me. Too much weight decreases the body's efficient use of insulin. I needed to think bigger thoughts, activate my volatiles, and get smaller. The food dreams stopped as I acted on my behaviorist's training, and followed premeditated principles, changing my eating habits. I began to slowly taste, eat selectively, and chew each bite twenty times. *Well, maybe twenty was an exaggeration. Ten seemed to get the job done.*

Once I banned eating on automatic pilot, I began feeling "new and improved." My official weight dropped by another twelve pounds and then plateaued. Refusing to get discouraged, I concentrated on blood sugar levels instead. They would let me know when I was eating properly and when I should feel guilty about what I was eating.

Even though the Cleveland area was shrouded with snow, I was still taking my bike for a hike most mornings and it was keeping my energy levels high. Dr. Carey said I was "improving." Measuring the last three months of blood sugar, the lab reading came back, *fair.* I had moved from *poor* to *fair* on my way to *good.*

"Keep doing what you are doing," she said. "And, you'll get to GOOD by your next visit in three months."

I'd keep to my morning practices of biking and journaling and be a finicky brat at the table. Feeling smug and filled with pride, the feeling didn't last long. There was always something else that I needed to change.

"I keep warning you about wearing heels and how important it is to cream your feet every night," said Dr. Carey.

My feet were dry, leathery and anything but soft. I used Excuse Number Five that always begins with a but.

"But they are always like this in winter."

"They don't have to be." She went on to discuss the merits of heavy-duty creams that were made especially for diabetics. I promised I'd cream them.

"And don't forget to throw out all your high heels," she said as she closed my chart.

"But, what would I wear with my dress suits?"

"Tennis shoes or tied oxfords would be great for your feet."

I looked at her feet. Dr. Carey wore white tennis shoes, which I hadn't noticed before. They looked fine with her white lab coat. *Maybe I'd start to wear a white lab coat.*

"Is there a dress code at your work?" she asked.

"No. But, high heels go with suits." *And being grown-up.*

"The men don't wear them with their suits and they have far fewer hammer toes than women." The discussion ended on that note. Tough to argue with that response. *Bend, Carole, bend.*

To celebrate moving into the *fair* range, I went to my favorite shoe store and didn't even look at any spiffy heels that made my shapely bicycle legs look longer. Well, I did sneak a peek but I only tried on a selection of suede loafers. I purchased a pair listed as dark chocolate. I chuckled to myself that they were better for me than a hot fudge sundae and a lot healthier, too. (I'd soon discover that I wore them because they felt so good on my feet even though I considered loafers unfashionable.) On the way to the cash register, I spotted a pair of black leather flats on the sale table. They would look a little smarter when I wanted to be "dressed up." I'd save one pair of high heels for special occasions even though the good doctor didn't want me to wear them at all. *Just a few times couldn't hurt, could it?*

Then I went to the video store and rented a mindless, new release. I didn't want a good drama or dark comedy that would engage my mind and make me think. I wanted fluff, laughter, and popcorn.

My blood sugar had bottomed out at 65 by the time that I arrived home making my body sweat. My hair was as wet as if I had been working out for an hour. My brain turned cranky. *Why couldn't my body eat fat and regulate itself?*

I poured raisin bran into a bowl and covered it with blue milk for a crunchy dinner. A quick fix was needed and I couldn't be bothered with preparing meat, salad, and vegetables. The cereal was tasty and sweet and I didn't feel deprived. *Hoo-Ray!* Who would have ever thought that I'd see cereal and my mom's blue milk as a satisfying dinner? I'd come a long way in changing my eating habits. I could feel my blood sugar rising as my mood mellowed with each spoonful. I didn't even mind much that my husband made himself pancakes, scrambled eggs, and sausage.

A "fair" lab reading, a bona fide weight loss, and a seal of approval from Dr. Carey. *No problems, right?*

Wrong, Carole, wrong. When I took my blood sugar reading the next morning, it was not at an eight-hour fasting level. It was soaring as if I had just eaten.

How could that be? I'd only had cereal for dinner. I purposely didn't have toast because I wanted popcorn with my video. I'd saved the calories and stuck to the carb combination choice. Well, I had cheated a little by cooking it in a tiny bit of oil because I didn't like the flat taste of air-popped popcorn.

Actually, I'd made myself a fry pan full of popcorn to share with my husband. He had declined a bowl because he didn't like the smell of the popcorn and was quite full of pancakes with maple syrup. *There are those volatiles again.* The heavenly scent of freshly popped corn was my trigger to eat more than my fair share. *And who was kidding whom? That fry pan was all for me or I'd have popped a second pan to have enough.*

For years I've agreed with everyone that popcorn was a good snack. If one was going to snack, it was better to do it with popcorn than with pizza, chocolate, cookies, peanuts, potato chips, or ice cream. But I was just kidding myself. It didn't matter what the food treat was; overindulging on any sweet or salty food led to trouble. After my satisfying popcorn binge, it shouldn't have been a surprise that my blood sugar level was not in the pre-meal, fasting range.

I was going to excuse myself from biking as a special dispensation because it was Friday and I'd had a good check-up. But diabetes was relentless and never went on holiday in my body. I needed to lower my blood sugar through medication and exercise. And, while doing so, I'd tow thoughts of popcorn, high heels, and the value of life.

The Parkway was virtually deserted. The sunrise was blooming pink against a steel winter sky. The bridge rails and trees formed black abstract designs against the winter morning. A flotilla of silent ducks was on one side of the bridge and two silent fishermen in hip waders were on the other. They were wet booted companions seeking open areas of water. No high heels there. They were kids at play and wait a minute, so was I. It felt good to be outside. Why had I even thought that it would be a reward to skip biking? Biking was a reward once I got off my duff and got moving.

Stopping on the bridge to soak in the gorgeous view, my eyes drifted to my feet, snug in high top, tennis shoes. I could feel my toes when I wiggled them. No damaged nerve endings yet.

Why was I being so resistive about giving up high heels? After all, I wasn't a long legged, Vegas showgirl. I was a social worker who wore tailored suits and jacket dresses. I did associate sensible, low heeled shoes with looking dowdy. I did not want to be seen as dull, prissy. If I wore my high tops to work, I would probably be seen as a tad eccentric. That'd be better than dowdy. I laughed at my fifty-something self.

So get over the fashion plate image of dressing with high heels. Wear the loafers, high tops, or flats. Throw the high heels out. Make every day a special occasion for your feet.

I remembered learning to walk in my first heels and garter-belted hose. I strutted, liking how the heels and hose lengthened my legs and showed off my narrow ankles. I really towered over my short mother. Is that what's wearing high heels was all about? Did I symbolically feel superior, important? Did I feel like I had showgirl potential in heels?

I needed to discover a fashionable body image for myself even though I could never look like my petite mother. That would be truly grown-up! *Maybe that was part of my struggle. I looked like Dad's side of the family and never accepted that my looks could ever be as pretty as my mom's were. Just as no one would ever say,"Carole eats like a bird," I had never been the cheerleader or dance floor jitterbug that mom had been. I was the bookworm, the administrator.*

I needed to have more fun with my image. I could start by adorning my feet in loafers, high tops, and flats. I wiggled my toes and counted them one by one.

This little piggy went biking. This little piggy wore high tops. This little piggy loved popcorn way too much. This little piggy's nose is very developed. This little piggy had a pen that writes the truth all the way home.

I rode on doing bike sprints and felt like a kid who had passed an important test and received a clean bill of health as a result. Radiating health is a good image. I was buoyant despite the morning's high blood sugar reading. Exercise would take it down.

Burn, popcorn, burn.

Popcorn had always been an old friend. In my childhood, it was a Sunday night treat along with the Ed Sullivan show. I could never get enough of the fragrant stuff. Often, I talked my mom into making another pan of it during the commercials. While it popped, she'd cut up red delicious apples into bite size wedges to work fruit into my diet.

"Too much popcorn isn't good for you. Learn moderation."

Yes, Mom. It has taken forever, but finally we're on the same page.

I needed to ban it from my shelves and stomach forever. If I snacked, the new me would eat celery, green pepper strips, raw cauliflower, carrot sticks. How many raw vegetables could anyone eat in one sitting? My total consumption would be less than my binge mountain of popcorn. I could keep watching the videos if I didn't snack on automatic pilot, or if I switched the accompanying snack to vegetables or gum. *I could practice chewing my cud.*

I groaned and then thought, *Maybe just one helping of popcorn would satisfy me.*

Then I thought back to my childhood. One serving didn't satisfy me then and it wouldn't now. I couldn't kid myself into believing that I have any restraint when it came to popcorn. Instead, give popcorn up.

Would I really give it up?

But I must change damaging habits and eat for a renewed self. Popcorn was no longer a comforting friend. Diabetes was my new food cop, or perhaps my body's adopted mom. It knew I needed a protective mother again, even if I didn't.

I'd say good-bye to popcorn. When I arrived home, I would fling my entire collection to the birds. The plumb golden ones that popped into a heavenly texture. The white kernels that popped light and fluffy. The cream colored kernels that taste so sweet. Throw out all kinds and all brands of popcorn.

On Saturday, I'd bag all the high heels and drop them off at Goodwill. I wanted to save my feet for later years. Maybe instead of the dreaded oxfords, I needed a rainbow wardrobe of sneakers. I could see me now, hand decorating them in sequins and pearls like many brides did wanting to save their feet on their wedding day. Didn't I want to save mine for every day, for the rest of my life?

The rosy sunrise faded as the sun rose flooding the Parkway with florescent light. I hiked my bike up the Detroit hill and out of the Valley Parkway leaving a trail of popcorn, high heels, and out-dated beliefs behind me.

I said a prayer of thanksgiving to the Creator of Life.

Thank you for getting me out into the elements to recreate whom you intended me to be. Continue to be patient with me because I'm as slow as the turtle when it comes to changing my thinking and my ways. But like the turtle, I plan to finish the race and with your help reach the GOOD blood sugar finish line, no matter how long it takes me. Belief conditions experience, and experience then strengthens the belief. What I believe, I experience. Amen.

*"You can't depend on your eyes when your
imagination is out of focus."*
—Mark Twain

Chapter Thirteen...At the Borderline: Ansel, Mary, & Mom

The ice bubble surface of the trail popped under the wheels of my bike like the red rolls of cap gun tapes of my childhood. Pop. Pop. Pop. The sound delighted me. Who would have thought at age fifty that I, the Queen of Comfort, would still be biking on a blustery Saturday at 6:30 a.m.? The parkway was deserted on this winter morning with the exception of a club pack of Roadrunners chattering down the all-purpose trail. Once they passed me, the trail was again filled with blissful solitude. It felt good to be alone, letting the day unfold. The sun was rising east of the river, casting growing shades of winter light on the woodland trail. I felt one with the pathway as I biked to the popping sound underneath my wheels.

Ready or not, here I come. Carole is on the trail, not lolling around in her bed.

Reaching the Borderline Café at 7:10 a.m., the morning regulars were claiming their spots. I took my usual, two-seater table in the middle room but first I kidded with Donna Jean, a blonde who'd dubbed me, "The Writing Fool." Donna Jean sat in a black tank top and shorts, face still flushed from her morning gym workout, newspaper spread before her. She was a South Sea Island native compared to my Eskimo garb of a throat muffler, ski gloves, and an earflap hat that tied under my chin. Not about to let me get away with remarks about her *aloha* attire, she laughed at my winter layers, asking, "How can you move, let alone straddle a bike? You're gonna fall."

"If I do, I'd just bounce like a rubber ball!"

Un-layering, I ordered my usual scrambled eggs, tomato slices, English muffin, and decaf coffee. No juice, bacon, or fried potatoes appeared at my table. The day stretched ahead and was mine to use/

abuse. My only plan was to cocoon, relax, and copy passages into my journal from Ann Linnea's narrative in *Deep Water Passage*. Ann Linnea kayaked 1200 miles around Lake Superior as a life challenge for herself. She set this goal because she said she learned best through body/action. She had wanted new learning, new directions.

"My whole life had been about pushing. Pushing to get good grades, a good job, a good home, good children. I couldn't push anymore. I just had to stay still, to keep up with nobody but myself. "

I certainly could identify with Linnea's journey. My morning ritual of mind and body practices were about keeping up with myself through rediscovering an active, out-of-doors self and writing about my thoughts afterwards. I was still working on learning to stay still and not worry how my life was stacking up or if I could ever afford to retire.

Several days into her trip, Ann Linnea had been resting even though she had wanted to keep going. But listening to her body she realized that she needed a break from paddling. Sitting still, a magnificent caribou appeared out of the woods unaware of her human presence. After drinking his fill of the icy blue water, he merged back into the trees.

"I resumed paddling. Slower now. Reminded once again that every moment holds the potential for magic. That those of too directed purpose can often pass by greater purpose."

I didn't want to miss the caribou magic either. As a new soul mate, Ann Linnea was reinforcing my desire to learn stillness as was Andrew Wyeth in his message to take it abroad and tow it awhile while reflecting on which direction I wanted to take in the second half of my life.

My husband of twenty-five years was pleased that I was "playing" as he often complained that I didn't take time to play. When asked to define "play," he had meant, "not working all the time," "having fun," and "interactive sports." While it's true I didn't play hockey, shoot hoops, seldom spiked a volleyball, golfed, or roller-bladed, I did "play" now. After all, it was Saturday and I wasn't at work, but enjoying the woods. Writing about his complaint in my journal, I think what my husband really meant was that before Vegas, I'd lost my sense of playfulness, the capacity to be surprised. I had been overly serious, intent on getting the children through college, making enough money, being a good daughter and helpmate, rather than relishing my days. Looking backwards, I could see that he'd been right. My senses had dulled. Work, however satisfying, was work. And, I'd stopped writing, something that had always produced natural highs within.

Now I was writing again for pleasure, learning the texture of my mind through journaling. But I wanted to expand my play beyond writing, greedy person that I was. Or was it the deprived bohemian child within that needed more? Maybe this shift in perspective would produce a breakthrough. I just knew that the starved, greedy me needed a new kind of magic like the caribou or the reign of golden yellow maples that had slowed me down to a state of wonder, laughter bubbling up from within. My bike hikes were a good beginning, but I wanted more caribou magic. But paddling a kayak 1200 miles wasn't going to be my way of finding it.

Sipping my second cup of decaf at the Borderline, the Roadrunners were arriving to discuss times, shoes, and the day's run. No one was talking about being one with nature, or the slant of the morning sun illuminating tree limbs. I was hooked on my new form of solitary exercise. My video workout tapes that emphasized movement and endurance were now just a test of endurance to continue. I was tired of the music and the people on the screen screeching instructions. These tapes reminded me of the piano metronome of my childhood. It never became my rhythm. It was someone else's beat. I preferred the wind in the trees and bird whistles. As I tuned out the running crowd and their bragging spirits, I knew that I didn't want to run anymore with the usual crowd. I certainly identified with Ann Linnea about pushing, pushing, and pushing oneself some more. What did I want to do instead?

I knew I was asking the right questions and didn't have to find instant answers. Writing and biking were a good beginning. I relaxed, and the Ansel Adams's southwestern photographs in *The Mural Project 1941-1942* hanging on the north wall of the Borderline came into focus. The image of the Taos Pueblo Church, New Mexico invited me to enter inside as Ansel Adams had centered and captured the entrance outlined in dark eye shadow, void of people. My kind of place to match my reflective mood today. A Mesa Verde photo had captured the intricate textures of an empty cliff dwelling, what living there had been like.

I sighed, envious. I wished I could be an Ansel Adams traveling the Southwest capturing the magic of "PLACE."

But wait, Carole. You could play with your Vegas camera in the Valley Parkway that you've come to love capturing the magic that PLACE.

I could, couldn't I?

I could pretend to be Ansel's eyes and practice being still, focused, quiet. Although I'd put aside the fantasy of becoming a photojournalist, I still carried my Vegas camera in my backpack. I'd now put it in a deep jacket pocket, loaded, and ready to use on my bike rides.

Excited, I thought of the photos that I had already missed, just like the fishermen do, spinning yarns about the ones that got away. But I hadn't even tried to lure the pictures into focus because I lacked the audacity and skills to capture what I was seeing and feeling. Or, could I have caught the color of the golden yellow sanctuary of reigning maple leaves, the circling of the crows, or an awesome sky at dawn? Pushing the decaf aside, I sipped at a glass of iced water, my imagination growing hot. These 35mm photos would be trigger memories of the Parkway's many healing and magical gifts. Even if I couldn't catch what moved me, the photos would be souvenirs of the trail. Photo journaling would just be another way besides words to freeze-frame myself and really see the interior journey. They'd become my valley eyeglasses.

As I journaled some more, a childhood memory crept onto the page. I was in the first grade, sitting at my desk in the back of the classroom, so placed because of my height and excellent deportment. Being a model student who liked learning, I was rewarded with good grades and the perk of sitting quietly at a rear window seat. So when I complained to my teacher that I couldn't see the blackboard, she paid attention. My mother was phoned that very day and, fretting, she took me after school to the eye doctor.

"Wouldn't I have noticed if Carole had vision problems?"

"Not necessarily. But by the very shape of her eyes, I can tell that she does," said the doctor.

What shape was that? I wondered, but too afraid to ask. Didn't I see like other people? How odd was that? Followed by the question, How odd was I?

Two days later I had a pair of clear plastic eyeglasses because my mother found them less pronounced than the tortoise shell glasses that I'd wanted. But as an adult and thinking back on those first glasses, I think the choice of which glasses was made more for a mother who was in shock and didn't accept that I needed glasses. Both she and my father had been college athletes who enjoyed the gift of excellent vision. Where had my poor vision come from? It wasn't on the genetic tree, but neither had diabetes been there. Feeling guilty, even when it wasn't anybody's fault, only leads one to nowhere.

Driving home from the optical store, I sat in the back seat of the car amazed at what I was seeing. Things were different than I had thought. For instance, I had always thought that leaves on the tall oaks were a part of a mass. When autumn arrived, it had been my belief that the wind ripped them off from a whole leaf fabric. That's why they floated to the ground jagged, torn, and brown. I looked in wonderment at individual oak leaves framed against the sky as part of the revised world that was before me. Upon hearing this discovery, my mother fretted some more, but never had to remind me to wear my glasses.

Bike riding combined with journaling was like putting on that first pair of glasses. If I added photography to my morning practices, just think of what I might discover. "The Writing Fool" may also become "The Photo Fool." I'd be a photojournalist yet; whose disease of diabetes forced a revisioning of who I was and what I saw in the world around me. My diabetes called for new eyes to put life into focus. I needed to see more clearly where I was going. The Vegas camera would be like new glasses slowing me down to the catch the caribou magic of the Valley Parkway and reinventing the playful me. I could be buddies with nature artists, Ansel Adams, Georgia O'Keeffe, and Jim Brandenburg.

Let's not get carried away, Carole.

Why not?

Indeed, why not? Caribou magic was waiting for me.

I began a photo portfolio labeled, "The Valley Parkway Project." A year later, I had a dozen or so images that spoke volumes to me. A solitary duck floated blissfully on the blue Monet rocks of the early morning riverbed. A deer camouflaged by a thicket of winter woods was labeled as the a-mazing deer. Sunlight streamed through the upraised arms of a tree. It became the "Praise Be Tree" and I watched for its blessings on morning bike rides. Concentrating on photographing trilliums lying prone in a field, I looked up and made eye contact with a young male deer sprouting velvet antlers. Velvet antlers became a favorite image.

I was growing in new directions. Playing at photography was such fun. But Ansel, Georgia, and Jim didn't need to worry, I was just playing, but I felt linked to them in passion. So if photography was my passionate play, writing became my serious avocation.

Between journaling and attending writing workshops, the theme of loss kept pushing up through the field of words. Loss of smooth-skinned legs blemished by aging—corded arteries and starburst veins. Loss of a devoted mom—feeling orphaned at fifty, childhood home sold and gone forever except in memory. Loss of Mary—my backyard neighbor and confidant to cancer, the disease eating through my generation of friends. My journal pages reeled from jottings of losses.

Was this what the second half of life was all about? Would I need a thicker philosophy to blanch the sorrow? I could keep my old legs covered, pretend to be a photojournalist, and send prayers asking for sustenance from Mom and Mary.

Mom and Mary were irreplaceable and both had enlivened and brightened the first half of my life. Both had taught me that gifts often come disguised. Maybe it took a half a lifetime to recognize a perfect gift for what it really was. Or, maybe I was just a slow learner. For instance, there was always the table story standing before me as a reminder.

On my eleventh birthday, my mother papered my bedroom with roses climbing on a white trellis into an endless sky. A pink and blue, pinwheel quilt emerged from her Singer sewing machine. White eyelet curtains drifted around the windows making soft shadow notes. But where there should have been a writing desk, a painted dressing table skirted in white eyelet with blue satin ribbons hugged a mirrored wall niche. It was a bedroom my mother would have swooned over as a young girl. It was a room my girlfriends pronounced as "Perfect." It was a room that was no longer me.

"Quite a showpiece, Mom." What I really wanted to say was, "What happened to the mother who often excused me from chores when I was scribbling into a notebook?"

This mother defended me to grandmother, saying, "Carole's going to write a book someday." Wouldn't this mother put a proper desk, and not a dressing table, in this daughter's room?

Since there wasn't a desk, I pushed the falderal aside and stacked paper and pens on the dressing table's glass surface. This put a crack in my mother's support of my writing career.

"Stop. You'll scratch the glass." But I persisted hiding my pens and papers under the dressing table's skirt.

"You'll catch pens in the eyelet and tear it."

"I need a place to write, Mom. I can't write on my bed. An ink cartridge might explode on the new quilt. The floor's too hard. That leaves the dressing table."

My mother muttered that I didn't appreciate her talent and she went off for a smoke. I continued to use my dressing table as a desk and my mother continued to smoke.

That Christmas my mother squeezed a wall desk in the only space left in my storybook bedroom. This fold-up desk was hung with twelve-inch screws into a sliver of wall space between the entry and closet doors. As it had no legs, a chair was tucked flushed against it. Mom presented me with a box covered in leftover wallpaper to keep my writing stuff in.

"It's perfect, Mom." And it was because we both were happy with the room. Now I could disappear into my rose trellis world of make-believe, writing masterpieces without disturbing her's.

Years later, the contents of my childhood bedroom arrived at my doorstep as my parents were downsizing. I debated about hanging the wall desk in my bedroom but in the end I hung it in the basement. I put my rose trellis box on a closet shelf as a keepsake while shaking my head over the dressing table that had certainly seen better days. De-skirted, it was now a chipped, white skeleton of itself. I relegated the table to the neighborhood garage sale.

There Mary began examining its undersides while I ranted about its honored place in the bedroom of my youth. Mary purchased the table. At last, I thought, the table would be appreciated, because Mary's daughter loved frilly things. "With a new skirt, it will look lovely in Kathleen's room."

Giving me her Mona Lisa smile, Mary carted the table home.

Mary invited me over for tea and the table's grand debut. Kathleen did not get a dressing table with a swirling skirt. Instead under Mary's skillful hands, a black walnut table had emerged with boxy legs and two workable drawers that had once been nailed shut and bound tight with blue ribbons.

"Oh, Mary. Please, please give it back. How much do you want for refinishing it?"

"You can't have it. I've put a lot of me into this table and it's just perfect for Patrick. He's been wanting a desk."

"A desk," I sighed. My dressing table was a real writing place at last. I wanted to keep begging but kept my lips still for I cherished my friendship with Mary more.

"Besides," added Mary, "You already have three desks. How many do you need?"

I kicked myself all the way home. Mary was right. A desk was not the problem for I did have three desks scattered throughout the house. All were stacked with empty paper and pens waiting for the muse to arrive squeezed in-between work, chores, and family. Still I yearned for what I couldn't have—a perfect, black walnut writing table with tons of time to write.

Where was the mother who excused me from chores because her daughter was going to write a book someday? It was then that I knew who had to be this mother. I began getting up two hours before the household awakened letting my hand fill up the ruled pages.

When I nailed a book contract, I flew over to Mary's house.

"Guess you didn't need that old dressing table after all."

"No. I needed a kick in the behind from a friend."

Mary stood in line at a bookstore signing. Phoning me the next day, she said, "Your book is perfect."

Years passed and the children grew up. Life was crammed full when Mary was diagnosed with cancer. As a true warrior, she fought her disease but in the end it captured her. I knew she was at the finish line when I received a call from Mary telling me to come and reclaim the black walnut table. It seemed Patrick had outgrown it. Mary had to phone a second time before I reluctantly went. *Oh, how I didn't want to lose Mary.*

"How can I ever thank you for such a perfect gift?"

Mary hugged me and then I made us our last cup of tea together.

I didn't want to say goodbye to Mary but I did, and then carted the table home with tears streaming down my cheeks. I still wanted the table, but I didn't want it. It would take awhile to look at it with clear eyes.

Well, Mom and Mary were both gone now, but the table remained. The black walnut swirls and whorls resonated in my bedroom so placed reminding me of where I came from and where I still yearned to go. On bad days, when my inner critic told me, *Give it up. This is useless,* I thought about turning my perfect desk back into a dressing table.

But I wouldn't, because I now knew what a perfect gift was. This gift was family and friends who deeply cared and believed in me. Everyone, but especially the stubborn me, needed confidants and encouragement no matter what happened. So I'd believe in myself even when I was stuck and stammered on paper. It was then that I needed the black walnut table the most, my talisman standing by a window that fluttered with white eyelet curtains.

Standing in my room, I felt close to Mom and Mary, closer than visiting them in a cemetery. Hugging my journal, they were now captured in words for me to visit and revisit. As long as I lived, they were with me. Oh, how I missed them.

"Not everything has a name. Some things lead us into a realm beyond words. By means of art we are sometimes sent—dimly, briefly—revelations unattainable by reason."
—Alexander Solzhenitsyn

Chapter Fourteen...A Call for Artists

I didn't know that I was missing an essential energy exchange with unknown, necessary friends. After all, I had friends and didn't have enough time to spend with them as it was. Combining healthy doses of protected solitude for writing and shooting pictures while working a demanding, sixty-hour workweek made me draw a line about joining anything.

At the dietician's urging, I attended the diabetic support group at the local hospital and it scared me into paying attention to my new companion of Type 2 Diabetes. But I didn't go back, because I couldn't yet see the amputations, walkers, and wheelchairs of my possible future without gasping for air, terrified. The social hour after the talk was a genteel tea party with plates of fresh fruit. I couldn't bear to stand there being accepting and gracious. Instead, I went screaming into the parking lot and drove away from these diabetic comrades as fast as I could go.

Lindsey, a good friend, had urged me to take *The Artist Way* course being offered at church. But like other offers of yoga, prayer groups, hiking, bird watching, aquatic aerobics, book discussions, or computer clubs, I excused myself despite an interest in those activities.

"I just can't commit or rush to one more meeting. I collapse after work."

As good friends do, Lindsey understood and accepted my refusal to book Tuesday evenings with *The Artist Way*. However, getting immersed in the course, she dropped off a copy of Julia Cameron's book, urging me to read it.

I didn't get to it right away, but when I did my mind leapt with ideas and questions. Here was a parallel path for getting in touch with oneself. Julia did three morning pages of journaling and made weekly, solo artist dates with herself. I found myself writing back to this new companion in my journal pages about my daily biking date with nature and photojournaling. I thanked my friend, Lindsey, for giving me such a gift of validation, words to label self-discoveries (morning pages and artist dates), and revelations revealed by another's journey.

So when Lindsey brought me a flyer calling for workshop presenters for an *Artist Way* Retreat to be held in Lakeside, Ohio, I submitted a proposal to teach *Point & Shoot Photography*.

My friend, Mary, of the rescued writing table had always wanted to open a bed and breakfast in Lakeside. This gated community hugged the shoreline of Lake Erie, two hours west of Cleveland. I just knew if Mary had loved Lakeside, I would find a part of what I loved about Mary there. And, if I shared my photoplay, I would really see Lakeside.

Once accepted as a speaker, I organized my workshop around what I considered the three essential elements of a good talk. These elements are: passionate stories out of the presenter's experience, a handout of tips on actual techniques, and an experiential interaction with the material presented.

And, if I was really truthful about my motivation to present, I did so for the simple fact that I wanted my tuition waived to cut down on the expense of attending. I was slowly absorbing the bartering principles learned from a Vegas shopgirl. However, it later turned out that it would have been far cheaper to go as a participant because of what the workshop spawned within me. But I didn't know about those consequences at the time. Probably just as well that I didn't or I might have run screaming, "I'm not ready yet."

Unaware of what laid in wait for me, I fooled around with my photographs. The workshop forced-bloomed them into an end product of greeting cards. I made several of my best Valley Parkway Project images into *gifts given to me to give* to the participants. Call it a bribe or a reward for taking the workshop, I wasn't going empty-handed.

I also packed up photos that didn't work, taken the same day of a prized picture, to discuss what worked and why. I rationalized that I could teach this workshop if everyone saw my photo art as play. The images were unplanned and spontaneously taken. I took whatever got caught in my eye during my morning rides through the Valley Parkway. My whole body hummed when I stopped, unleashed my camera, and followed the light. For the workshop, I chose: the long back of the heron fishing along the edge of the Rocky River; a squirrel scrambling up a blazing-golden oak; a Monet duck serenely paddling amongst blue slate rocks; the a-mazing deer eyeing me from behind a thicket of trees; one red leaf clinging to a huge maple against a winter blue sky.

These photos were presents given to me. After all, I had no art institute training. With my Vegas purchased camera, I was being given "winning" reminders of the beauty that surrounded me if I only took the time to look. Julia Cameron called this the gift of "paying attention," finding joy in the everyday details of life. By offering a "point and shoot" workshop, I made a play date with other seekers of beauty.

The workshop went more than well, taking on a life of its own. I opened with eleven participants pouring over a varied collection of photographs in books, calendars, and postcards. Images hooked us all. After this immersion into photos, we went around the circle introducing ourselves through our choices. Their different selections made us think and connect with one another on more than a superficial level. A couple of choices really resonated inside of me.

A trainer of thoroughbred horses held up a photo of a tree blurred by snow that I'd never looked at twice because I was drawn to clarity and color. Although it was a color photograph, the blurred tree was gray and black in a sea of wispy white snow.

"I love being out in this kind of snow. It's soft, first snow. It's not slippery and there is a hush in the air. A sacred hush. On my horse, I feel alone, but not alone. It's hard to explain."

But she had because I knew what she was speaking about. I'd biked in this snow through the Valley Parkway. I looked at the photo again appreciating how photos trigger more than memories. They touch emotions, which we can then put into words.

The owner of the Bed & Breakfast where we were staying held up a picture of an old table with a bucket of wild flowers. The flowers were the focal point of a very busy, yet inviting photo, a kaleidoscope of random colors and shapes.

"I don't like the polished country look. I like the real country, cluttered look."

Looking about me, I saw that her B & B had a whimsical, crazy quilt quality that worked. Our hostess had an uncanny, artistic knack for spillages of unexpected eye treats. Her inn was filled with photo opportunities. I was particularly drawn to a bird's nest with three eggs and a spray of flowers gracing a nearby corner table.

A librarian, the color of chalk, with wispy, blonde hair chose a black & white photo of an empty table and chairs on a stone patio overlooking a flat sea. "I'd like to sit there for a week doing nothing." We all identified with that wish. She sighed and looked again at her choice adding, "That's bizarre. I didn't see the lizard crawling on the table and what it might mean to me, but I still choose this photo."

The lizard added interest to this otherwise picture perfect view hinting that all was not as it seemed. Or perhaps, that life was ultimately a big paradox.

Two participants chose the same photo featuring a night-time ocean, illuminated by a spectacular, moonbeam of light breaking through the heavens and hitting the water like a spotlight. Excited by this phenomenal shot of nature, they called it, *God's Slide*. We talked about "the gift" of such an artistic encounter. Carrying a small camera can capture such unplanned, God Moments. Even if the shot did not turn out as elegant as the one before us, the mind could return to the encounter with the nudge of a documented reminder.

Each photo choice was a revelation of communion with each other. As we talked, we drew close seeking understanding. Finally, we came to the last participant, Sandy, whose husky voice startled me because it sounded exactly like my friend Mary's. Sandy held up a photo of a gray wall of mountain rocks. Dwarfed by this sheer face of rock, was a pair of red hooded monks sitting in a cave in the far right corner.

"This photo speaks to me. It reminds me to look beyond myself and see the larger perspective." *I had been drawn to Lakeside because Mary loved it. Was Mary in the room, reincarnated? My body trembled in response.*

Asking the group to discuss this photo's composition, I kept hearing Mary's voice ringing in my ears. "Look beyond the dressing table, outside of yourself."

The workshop continued as we shifted to looking at my documented snapshots and the contrasted *gift* shots. We saw together what worked as I had played with the camera. One example was a shot of an ordinary view of a hibiscus bush and another of the street sign where it was taken for later reference. Then I showed them a card of just two mallow hibiscus hugging, blushing in full-faced beauty, a la Georgia O'Keeffe.

A former photography major clapped her hands and said, "The first two are just snapshots." She continued, saying that she had stopped taking pictures because of her need for perfection and a perceived lack of time to set-up the shots she wanted. "The third shot is ART! By showing us all three and how photography can be playful, I feel liberated. Thank you. Oh, how can I ever thank you!"

Overwhelmed by the release she was experiencing, I took a deep breath and was glad of my therapy training. I kept still, allowing her to fully experience her joy. I'd never expected any awakenings to happen in this puny workshop on *Point and Shoot Photography*. It was the last response I'd expected. After all, I'd just been playing, not working. Then I heard Mary's voice again, now inside of me. *Are you sure that you're only playing?*

It was time to move the workshop into the experiential photo walk about Lakeside. The cottages had white trellis gardens, companion chairs arranged to sit, talk, or read. Lacy bric-a-brac outlined doorways, windows, and fences. Everywhere we looked, there was a photo waiting to be snapped. We discovered seven, different angel statues and I felt blessed with each find. One angel had a crown of flowers and a patina that shimmered. Oak seeds adorned her shoulders. It was love at first sight. I'd found a guardian angel to hang over my desk.

The lake and its horizon were an inviting blue. Lakeside made our eyes delirious, dizzy with possibilities as we took pictures of what spoke to us. The photography major was lying on the ground getting shadows of bikes & bike racks. Staying intrigued with shadows, she captured herself taking a picture in a full-sized, shadow that spoke volumes to and about her. *Once home, I wondered would she emerge from the shadows and practice her art? For that matter, would I? I was having a hard time thinking of my photography as art. I was just snapping pictures, wasn't I? Some were just better than others.*

Unwinding over a cup of tea by myself after the workshop, a primitive poem took shape.

Hatchlings

Three blue eggs
In a nest,
Perfect orbs,
Unhatched.
Nestled like Moses
In a boat of woven
Bulrushes and caulked mud,
An intricate, sturdy craft
Holding dreams.
Delicate,
White blossoms

Kiss the bow.
Surely not
A funeral
Barge?
Mourning
Unborn
Hatchlings
Singing
New songs!
Breathe.
Blow the spark of life
Into blazing dreams.

Up before dawn the next morning, I filled my journal with snips of the full weekend experience of tomato poetry, drumming, storytelling, photography, artist dates, and morning pages—and found a missing piece of myself. Artists all, we sang circling songs of homecoming to each other. We rejoiced in the gift of creativity and the shifts in perspective that it offered us. Whatever losses I'd experience in the second half of life, I now knew that I'd have to have artistic friends and art itself to shoulder personal earthquakes when my place on this ground shifted under me.

Energized, I closed my journal and picked up my camera. I followed the blooming light to see the sun rise over Lake Erie. Other participants were up early scattered on solitary benches or walking. Everyone was respectful of the dawn pursuits of reading a book, journaling, or just breathing in the quiet of a Lakeside morning. As the Retreat was booked in the off-season, there were no crowds, traffic, or restaurants open. Only the lone, white security car made its punctual rounds. I shot three rolls of film. I caught the sun's rays washing gold over every wave, tree, and the pink center of a cabbage rose.

Filled with beauty, I was startled, yet comforted to hear Mary's husky voice again. But, it was her double, Sandy who had caught up with me to walk to breakfast.

"You are God's artist. You are capturing his landscape through your focus on nature. You have inspired me." She was silent for a few minutes and then added, "You owe it to yourself and others to share this gift. When I get home, I'm going to talk to a gallery owner that I know. I'm sure she'll want to carry your cards."

"Thank you." It was all I could say at the time. I was moved by her belief in me, but I wouldn't hold my breath because galleries only carried images made by real photographers. And the cards had only been made to share in the workshop. Strangers wouldn't want to pay money for them.

However, surrounding oneself with artists was like the park's wind pushing me into spots of beauty. Once home, I agreed to teach *The Artist Way* in an artist cooperative that began to sell my cards to strangers. Afterwards, the class took on a life of its own as a cluster support group of which I became a lifelong member. I'd discovered that artists needed not only huge doses of solitude, but they also needed to rub viewpoints with other creatives, regardless of artistic persuasion. I'd found my missing support group that would further heal me inside out without me running screaming into the parking lot. Playing, working, and sharing art would make me whole. After all, as Julia Cameron says, "God loves an artist." *And so do I. Therefore, I must become one because they are my true tribe.*

"If you have made mistakes...there is always another chance for you...you may have a fresh start any moment you choose, for this thing we call 'failure' is not the falling down, but the staying down."
—Mary Pickford

Chapter Fifteen...Falling Down

The city streets were weepy with salt, but no longer slippery. I should have stayed on them but thought I'd be safer in the pre-dawn darkness on the bike trail rather than on the Valley Parkway Road. Pumping my wheels up over the curb onto the trail, I hit black ice. Spinning out-of-control, my whirling front tire shimmied up and bucked me off. Smack. I landed hard on my back and head. Racked with pain, I lay wondering if I could get up. The biking kid in me felt every inch of her fifty-something body.

"Are you okay?" The driver of a gray van had pulled over. "I have a cell phone."

I waved him off. "Thanks for stopping, but I don't think anything's broken. I'm just gonna rest for a minute. "

He didn't seem convinced and didn't leave.

I forced myself to a sitting position and pasted a smile on my face. "I'm okay, just embarrassed." Again I assured him that I was all right.

My potential benefactor left. Unobserved, I dragged up my bike with me as I stood on trembling legs. I wobble-walked for a few feet, then mounted my bike, and rode slowly home. In the safety of my house, I breathed a sigh of relief. No ambulances with flashing red lights had been needed for this crazy, fifty-something lady. Hanging up my white parka, I took off my biking helmet. It broke in two in my hands. That undid me. I sat on the basement steps, fell apart, and sobbed. *What if I hadn't been wearing it? Humpty-Dumpty and I would have had lots in common. I thanked Mom, Mary, and the Lord for bike helmets.*

My back was not as fortunate as my head. It throbbed. I took a hot shower and felt better. I went to work. *Was I crazy? Had my head been affected after all?* I think I was in shock and stayed in shock until I arrived home and found I couldn't stretch out on my bed. *Why hadn't I gone to the doctor's office? Why didn't I go to the Emergency Room now?*

My husband and I decided I'd probably broken a rib or two. He thought maybe I should get a medical opinion, but he agreed with me that they'd probably just tape it. I didn't go, not wanting a lecture on the foolishness of a fifty-year-old biking in winter.

I gave up bike riding and brought popcorn into the house labeling it as therapeutic. It was just a matter of time before I became the Video Queen again. I was lost.

Three weeks after *the fall*, I was cranky, out of sorts. Unable to lie flat, I'd taken to sleeping in the family room recliner. *What had I been thinking? That I was still eleven and flexible? That I could really change my sedentary ways at age 50? Could I really teach this dog new tricks? Who was I kidding? Only myself, it seemed.*

My husband suggested that we could walk after dinner for exercise.

I gave him the evil eye. I didn't want to walk. *Thank you very much.* I wanted to ride my bike and be eleven again, or do nothing else. Plus, unable to bear the weight of my backpack, I missed the saddlebags on my bike to carry journals, pens, and my Vegas camera. My morning routines were trashed. I remained inflexible in more ways than not being able to lie flat on my back. I even stopped weighing myself. A sure sign that I was putting on weight.

Such was my *pity party* mood when I drove in tight-fitting clothes to Mohigan State Park for a three-day, state mandatory training on adoption. I think my husband was relieved to have my foul mood gone for a few days.

I'd been pleased that at least the state trainer giving the certification was a gifted workshop leader, Denise Goodman, Ph.D. She'd be the saving grace for this "know-it-all" social worker who truly believed she'd heard it all before.

Dr. Goodman didn't disappoint me. She was funny, outrageous, and passionate about the beautiful 1800 children waiting for adoption in the Ohio public child welfare system.

"We work for the children. We aren't doing a good enough job for Ohio's legally free children waiting for a forever family. That forever family may never come if we don't get a move on."

Denise clicked along at a fast pace challenging us to be "recovering assumers." We assume that adoptive parents heard what we said about the disturbing behaviors of the sexually abused child when these parents were focused elsewhere. Instead of listening to the facts, they were perhaps thinking about how much the child's picture reminded them of a cherished aunt. We assumed they heard the provocative, angry, self-abusive behaviors that these children often exhibited rather than thinking that all it took was a good heart and love to raise these kids.

As usual, Denise was crashing down participant barriers. And if you weren't paying attention or talking to a neighbor, a sponge ball might get thrown in your face in Denise's workshop. What I needed was someone to throw a sponge ball at my mouth when I rudely assumed that my diabetic body could handle donuts and coffee, standard workshop fare.

But what I liked best about Denise's training style was that she not only demanded attention and challenged me to learn something; she also offered solutions. She didn't pull apart old beliefs and behaviors without giving a framework to use the new learning. And, that's how I came to learn about "*The Prediction Path.*"

Denise and some Toledo colleagues had worked out a tool to help parents think about a specific child's challenging behaviors, when these behaviors might surface, and how to handle these behaviors at different ages and stages of development. Such preparation can prevent feeling out-of-control, taking the behavior personally, and generally feeling helpless. Denise said she wanted parents to view unhealthy behaviors not as "problems" which have to be tolerated but as "needs" that have solutions. *The Prediction Path* proved to be a marvelous tool to organize information and prepare caregivers for foreseeable behaviors of "special needs" children.

After a night of deep sleep with my unconscious sifting through the rich composts of workshop learning's, I awakened early, eager to once again journal. Voila! Why couldn't I create "Carole's Diabetic Prediction Path" (CDPP) to address my own special needs. It would protect me from falling back into bad habits. Such a tool would help me to think of diabetes not as a problem to be endured but as my body's need to get healthy. I could improve on my caregiver skills to myself.

"Kabam! Thank you, Denise!"

My mind shifted into a spinning hum. I had a new way to address my diabetes using planned interventions that built upon my strengths and identified my Achilles heels. I modified the format of "The Prediction Path" for my use. I would create one page per each identified behavior challenge and keep adding to this pathway as I went along my journey.

Carole's Diabetic Prediction Path Framework (CDPP) consists of four columns labeled as **Trigger, Intervention, Do Now, Life-Long.** The Trigger is a feeling or action that sets off a chain reaction. What does this feeling signify or when did this behavior start? What significant tapes keep playing in the mind or body? Put identified behavior/feeling in this first column. Journal about this topic until some understanding is gained about what's going on.

The Intervention involves asking what action, affirmation, or therapeutic healing is needed. Even if I haven't figured out what's behind the identified trigger, I can begin to act differently to change the re-action. Make a list of steps needed or choices.

Do Now is choosing to act *immediately,* not letting the trigger take over; to change how I'm feeling. This step builds confidence in being able to change. Place right now action steps in this column.

Life-Long recognizes my Achilles' Heels. I know what depletes my life energies. Begin to predict when triggers will happen and what I need to do when they happen. Choose to energize myself instead.

Once I had the framework, I tried out Carole's Diabetic Prediction Path (CDPP).

Behavior / Feeling Challenge: A Setback

Trigger	Intervention	Do Now	Life-Long
Break a rib biking.	Healing time needed.	*Baby* self.	If patient, will heal. Just seems *forever.*
	Follow routine minus the biking.	Can still write. Can still have breakfast out.	Resume old habit biking) when healed.
Any crisis.	Establish needed new habits.	Do what can do that's healthy.	Be open to new ways, paths.
	Put emergency shelf together.	Organize non-food treats / rewards. Pick one.	ER supplies take care of *crazies.* Keep it stocked.

I developed an emergency (ER) shelf when I was new to parenting. When my head was whirling from kid breakdowns, I'd go to the ER shelf. There I'd find not only star-studded Band-Aids, but a whole deck of cards to play matching numbers, a roll of quarters to play hooky with the kids by getting on a local bus, coupons for area recreation, the pin to blow up the kick ball, big chalk to draw pictures or a hopscotch grid, music to dance around and get happy. What I needed now was a diabetic ER shelf for a fifty-year-old child. I'd stock it with bubble bath, a roll of quarters to ride the bus, gift certificates to area businesses, batteries and film for my camera, fine line pens, a blank journal, music inspiring contemplation, and music to dance around and get happy.

I tried a couple more diabetic challenges of mine.

Behavior / Feeling Challenge: Eating As A Reward

Trigger	Intervention	Do Now	Life-Long
1. **Long day** tiredness.	1. Nap. Go for bike ride for energy, stress release.	1.Lay down. Repeat after me, "Food is not the answer." Drink water.	1. Recognize eating as not pick-me-up or reward for a diabetic.
2. **Celebration**	2. Don't build around a meal. Focus on the Joy you are feeling.	2. Choose a different reward. Sing. Dance.	2. Keep a list of rewards handy. Do anything but eat large. Buy a trinket!
3. **Leisure** When eating out, don't use as an excuse to splurge.	3. Take an Artist Date. Plan some Fun that doesn't involve eating.	3. Socialize. Journal. When writing in cafes, sip tea, coffee. Order a fresh fruit plate.	3. Use restaurants as a support, not the road to ruin. Order two appetizers instead of four course meal.

Behavior / Feeling Challenge: Food Can't Manage Feelings, Losses, & Changes

Trigger	Intervention	Do Now	Life-Long
1. **When upset.** Identify what feeling.	1. Soothe self with writing.	1. Recognize losses.	1. Pray for peace, grace.
2. **Awareness** of anniversary dates of losses.	2. Take a time-out to remember.	2. Examine feelings of sadness & anger.	2. Read book

3. Change creates losses & new openings.

3. Address needs created by accepting feelings.

3. Have a good cry.

3. Watch heart-felt video

4. Make a pampering date for self.

4. Bike to find legs & get endorphins in brain released.

4. *"Endure, and keep yourself for days of happiness."* –Eudora Welty

5. For grief work Write an essay. Start with, *I remember...* Second part, start with *But now....*

5. Visit a grave site and sit quietly for awhile. Seek communion with saints & spirits

5. Remember eating only offers a fleeting fullness; it doesn't fill me up

Pleased with Carole's Diabetic Prediction Path (CDPP), * I knew I'd keep crafting it as I learned best—from the inside out, by trial and error. I now had a road map with travel advisory tips to save myself from getting lost, discouraged, or frustrated as I trundled along and even broke a rib or two. When trapped in a flood of high blood sugar levels, I'd pull out this CDPP road map and use it as a bridge. I'd keep reviewing and revising it as my journey continued with my diabetic companion and realize that I had choices. Good choices.

* See Appendix for more identified behavior / feeling challenges using the CDPP.

Part Three

Second Story Woman...The Promised Land

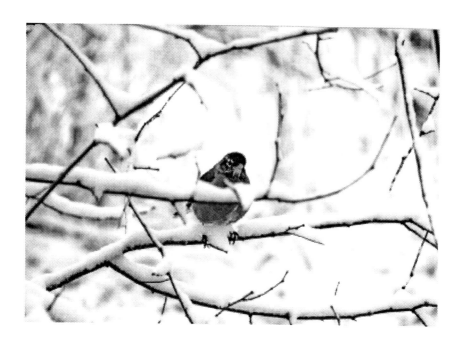

*"The walls of lack and delay now crumble away,
and I enter my Promised Land, under grace."*
—Florence Scovel Shinn

Chapter Sixteen...The Promised Land

"What do you mean, this is what's been decided?" I was indignant. I'd been commanded to drive to Columbus, agency state headquarters for an emergency budget meeting. The other regional directors sitting around the conference table were stirring their coffee, taking notes in their planners, or just staring off into space.

"Don't we get a say in this at all?" I asked.

"No, Carole. You don't," said Ruth, the State Director, straightening the papers in front of her. "But believe me. This wasn't an easy decision."

"Why don't you cut everyone's wage in the agency by 1 – 3 % to be re-instated when the budget turns around?" I continued my attack.

"In my experience, you lose your best people that way," said Mary Sue, glaring at me to shut up. "The best start looking for new jobs."

"But to lay off all of our part-time big brothers and sisters!" I felt like I'd been punched in the gut. "The foster children in our care will lose big time. Aren't we concerned about what's best for them?"

Ruth didn't want to go there. She drew back from the table as if I had punched her in the gut. Regaining her composure she said, "We had to balance the budget, Carole. This cut back is what's been decided. I'm thankful it only involves part-time staff." She held up her hand at me and continued. "With this adjustment, we should be okay again in four to seven months."

"We need to tap into the mental health funding stream in Cuyahoga County," said Mary Sue. "Carole, you can help me with getting certified to provide mental health services."

I didn't answer Mary Sue, afraid of what I might say.

And so on Friday, the very next day, all the big brothers and sisters received a pink slip in their paychecks. *We are sorry to inform you that due to budgetary constraints, you have been laid-off. Thank you for your service to children.* One by one, as they picked up their paychecks, the big brothers and sisters dropped in or phoned me. I commiserated with them. I hugged them and invited them to the next regional party. I didn't know what else to do or say.

I had plenty I wanted to say, but kept my anger to myself and instead tried to handle their anger. The case managers picked up some of the slack by putting in extra hours with the children to fill in. I, on the other hand, did help the agency obtain a new mental health funding stream for case management fees that would be in addition to the specialized child welfare room and board per diems. It took nearly a year, but finally every *i* was dotted and *t* crossed and our application was accepted. With new moneys, we were able to hire some of the big brothers and sisters back.

I breathed better but I was on empty. When would the next funding crisis occur? All the regions and states helped one another in times of financial crunches. I found excuses to not attend the monthly state meetings. Why bother if the regional directors weren't included in how to manage the budget? I felt I was just mouthing the party line to quiet the regional unrest. The agency felt financially as out of control as my diabetes had once been. The question became: Did I want to stay in this work environment?

I could stay put and magically believe that this wouldn't happen again. The best reason to stay was the hand-picked staff and foster families. There was a sense of family in this regional workplace. If I left, I knew I'd see myself as a deserter, even selfish. However, it came down to the fact that I no longer wanted to expend great personal effort to hold the region together and interpret yet one more state directive that I was powerless to change. I was ripe for plucking.

Sensing a change in me, the local child welfare agencies came recruiting. The two agencies that I was most interested in were very different. One was a *David* of an agency and the other was a *Goliath* agency with deep Cleveland, clinical roots. For the first time, I began to listen hard to their pitches.

The *Goliath* agency offered a $10,000 increase in pay. Sixty-hour work weeks were the norm. But hey, I certainly was used to working those hours. I could use my program development skills and be a big cheese in my hometown arena.

The *David* agency would match my current pay offering me an associate director position with a forty-hour work week as the norm. I wouldn't be in charge of a single program. Instead, I would be shoring up existing programs, concentrating on seeing that the children in care were well served. I'd personally worked well in the community with both the executive and other associate director.

I must admit that I struggled with stepping down. In the end, I asked myself whether I wanted money, a big title, and lots of work? Or, did I want a life plus social work satisfaction? It should be a no-brainer, right? Old messages of competition and the American way died hard in me.

However, I was proud of myself and the many lifestyle changes that I was making. I ultimately chose the *David* agency promising the executive director that I would work there for the next ten years. In doing so, I should have asked: *Are you giving me the same guarantee?* But that would be getting ahead of myself in this story of changing my life.

Realistically, it takes a full year to settle in and learn a new agency's policies and procedures. Meanwhile, building rapport and trust with the staff was difficult, especially since this staff thought I was on the scene to take over the agency. They gossiped amongst themselves.

Is Bob stepping down?

Is he sick? He has been looking pale lately and has lost a lot of weight.

Is he going to do more work for his church?

Is Carole being groomed to take over the agency?

They certainly weren't sure about what I was doing there. They watched me give up much of my community committee work. They remained puzzled.

As with any job change, my schedule and routines were in shambles. I did find, however, that my morning practices and prediction path (the CDPP) were not a fluke. They helped me keep my balance and perspective. But what motivated me the most was another choice that I was making in my personal life.

Our mortgage had been paid off. The children were through college. My husband had offered, "You don't have to work now. We could manage on my salary alone."

Andy was giving me a chance to write full-time and not wait for retirement as had been the plan. I could apply for my all-time favorite, drop-out position of dispensing tickets at the movie theatre. I'd have a little side income, see all the movies I wanted, and be surrounded by the wonderful auroma of popcorn. That would be heaven, albeit a little too much popcorn temptation. While I could certainly choose to coast and practice being dependent, it would be hard for me to do so, particularly since I was used to having my own checking account.

If I continued to work full-time in my profession, what would be my ultimate reward? What would I choose? I'd been pining for years for a house with a view, even if it meant a new thirty-year mortgage. It happened like this.

I'd been searching, long before biking, for a house with a view of the Cleveland Metroparks. When the children were growing up, I wanted to purchase a colonial house perched on the valley with a surrounding brick patio and white picket fence backyard with a western sky view.

"I talked to a naturalist in the park, Carole" said my husband. Andy didn't want to move and so he did his research. "The house is wonderful, but it's built on shale."

"So?" I asked, not really wanting to hear what was coming next.

"It'll fall into the Valley, some day," Andy explained. "It's why the basement is crooked now."

"So what?" I'd countered. "That's probably not going to happen in our lifetime."

"I'm not buying a house that's built on a hill of shale," was my husband's final word.

Once our kids had graduated from high school, my search broadened into other suburbs as I was no longer limited to staying in our school district. I found a jewel of a house on the other side of the Valley Parkway with an eastern view. It was set back on the lot. Andy agreed to put our family home up for sale and if it sold, we could purchase the new house. Our home didn't sell, but the jewel did.

The next house that I found on my morning bike rides was built into a hill. It had seven levels.

"Carole. Be practical. We are getting older, not younger," said Andy shaking his head.

"So?" I asked.

"Remember when you hurt your leg two weeks ago? How would you have ever managed all these stairs?"

"I'd put a hide-a-bed in the first floor den." I replied. "And in the long run, all these stairs would keep me young and fit."

My husband said, "No." Then he went out and bought me a six-foot by ten-foot, framed piece of stained glass of blue sky, clouds, and sea gulls that I'd been admiring in an antique store. It was lovely and we hung it in the front window of our family home.

Pleased with himself, Andy stood back and said. "Now you have your view."

Even so, I persisted in my search for a house overlooking the Cleveland Metroparks.

When I discovered the double-decker house, I was pushing my bike and myself up and out of the Valley Parkway on a steep road named Rockcliff Drive. Propping my bike against the metal guardrail at the top, I was breathing hard, my eyes on a bare armed tree reaching out into a spectacular sunrise. I rummaged into my pack for my camera.

A resident, coffee mug in hand, hurried out of her house. "Are you all right?"

"Yes." Straightening up, I waved my camera at the sky. "Isn't this sunrise gorgeous?"

Seeing that I was not having a heart attack and only shooting a few photos, she stood with me watching the dawn dance with swirling scarves of color until only the sky's blue dress was left.

"Thank you for your concern." I said.

"Quite all right." She nodded and went back inside probably saying to her family, "She was certainly huffing and puffing, but she wasn't doubled over in pain. She was searching in her backpack for a camera, not nitroglycerin pills."

I resumed biking thinking what a great street this would be to live on.

Then, I saw the house. Standing as an anchor at the end of the street waiting for me, was a brick, double-decker house with white, peeling lions guarding the front door and a "for sale" sign on its crab grass lawn. My first thought was: *I could be content living my days in this house.* It was an answer to my prayer for a house with a view and to the universal question, *If money were not a consideration, where would you like to live?*

My second thought was: *Too bad we couldn't afford this house.*

Seeing there was a restaurant parking lot next door, I rode down the blacktop lot to catch the valley view from the back of the house. The cliff's chin jutted out over the emerald necklace lands below. The Rocky River splashed over rocks and broken chunks of ice. Upraised tree arms celebrated the coming of spring. I had survived another winter, biking to the Borderline through the valley and understood this celebration by the trees. Thinking about what they would look like in the full dressed dance of fall, my excitement grew.

Dr. Carey would approve of this reward because it wasn't edible. I'd even carry a Miss Piggy lunch box to help pay for this reward. Just as I was thinking that it was too bad that we really couldn't afford this house, a huge chocolate Doberman lunged at the chain link fence barking, "Keep away." A leash line prevented his vault over the fence. I tore my eyes away from the valley view and looked closely at the back yard, which barely contained this horse of a dog. The lawn was a disaster being used as a dog run. A long leash was clipped to a wire strung from the bottom deck of the house to the first arm of a mammoth oak tree near the cliff's fenced edge. The yard was scruffy and needed a clean up from the many deposits of dog debris.

"Hmmm." If the inside was in as much disarray as the yard, maybe, just maybe, we could afford this house. I remembered reading in *Meditations, On the Monk Who Dwells in Daily Life,* a Thomas Moore story about a pilgrim, an abbot, and monks working on an abbey.

"It's good to see a monastery going up," said the pilgrim.

"They're tearing it down," said the abbot.

"Whatever for?" asked the pilgrim.

"So we can see the sun rise at dawn," said the abbot.

"To see the sunrise." This phrase reverberated throughout my body and I made an appointment to tour the house.

The inside of the Rockcliff House was more of a disaster. Starting in the basement, storage cubbyholes were overflowing. File boxes were everywhere in the owner's home office. They teetered on table edges and were scattered randomly throughout the basement. On the top floor, I couldn't see much of the floor either. Strewn clothes, empty pizza boxes, and clutter of the tenants made it impossible to see the condition of the carpet. The kitchen sink was clogged. A bucket was catching drippings from the plumbing elbow under the sink. The three T's of a friend's rental property made me tremble. Tenants, Toilets, and Trouble. However, the windows from the Florida room upstairs offered a redeeming view of the emerald necklace woods.

The downstairs apartment housed a husband, wife, the wife's mother recovering from a broken hip, and the dog. The Doberman pincher had jumped through the front bay window. Newly installed interior iron bars prevented that from happening again, but it didn't prevent this dog from having accidents in-doors in his favorite spots. It smelled like he'd been marking his territory as wolves did.

"Imagine it polished up," said the realtor as we picked our way through the yard.

Polished up, indeed. It needed to be torn down to see the sun rise. Even I couldn't stretch my imagination and see this double-decker house cleaned up and I have a pretty good imagination.

"I'll get back to you after I talk to my husband." But I knew better than to show this house to my husband or I might end up in probate court, my sanity in question.

Pushing the double-decker house aside in my head, I was glad that I was going on a little trip. While I was out of town, it would sell due to its prime location. It didn't matter what its condition was. Someone would buy and bulldoze it. And that would be that. I'd keep looking.

I'd planned a solo drive to my hometown of Clinton, Iowa. Dorothea had written at Christmastime inquiring if I would like the white dishes that she and Mabel had collected together. On my last trip to Iowa, I had helped Dorothea, executor of Mabel Foster's estate, lay Mabel to rest. Mabel and Mom had befriended each other in their first teaching positions and became life-long friends. Mabel had been the only babysitter that I'd ever known and she died of a heart attack a year after my mother's death. I hadn't been back to Iowa since.

Dorothea wanted someone to have the white dishes who would value them. For the life of me I couldn't remember the white dishes. As the recipient of much of Mabel's estate, I had her *Fostoria* hobnail dishes and her gold edged, *Limoges* China. For the life of me I couldn't picture the white dishes.

"You really need another set of dishes," jested my husband.

"I know. I know. But I want them anyway."

Andy asked, "What will you do with them?"

"Maybe when our sons settle down, they might like a complete set of dishes."

"They'd probably like a year's supply of paper plates instead."

I wrote Dorothea back that I would be honored to be the recipient of the white dishes, ignoring my husband's disapproval. I wasn't sure why I wanted them. I didn't think it was out of greed, at least I hoped not. I think the real reason was that it would give me a chance to visit Clinton again without husband or kids. I could take a good look around at the town that raised me.

Dorothea, with a three-prong cane, opened the door of her and Lillian's home. Wreathed in smiles of welcome, she greeted me just as she had at the bank when she'd been the executive secretary to the bank's president. Dorothea always used to take care of me personally when I cashed clerking paychecks received from VanAllen's Department Store.

We hugged and I felt dampness on my cheeks. Dorothea's formerly soft body was now all bones. Lillian's was even more so but she had always been angular and thin standing at her easel as one of the two high school art teachers. Lillian had a matching, three-prong cane.

"Our canes are a godsend," said Lillian. "Doors are opened for us and we can park close to wherever we're going. Just like royalty, the path is cleared."

"We don't go very far anymore," said Dorothea smiling.

"I'm glad I traveled when I was young," said Lillian. "I've traveled abroad and I've visited every state but Hawaii and Alaska. I have good memories. Do you travel much, Carole?"

"Can't say that I have. But I did go to Vegas recently. Does that count?"

"Fiddle-faddle. That's just a tinsel show in the desert," said Lillian. "You need to see Italy, France, Germany."

"I'd like to travel. Maybe I will now that the kids are raised."

They led the way to the dining room table where Lillian sat herself in the side chair closest to the window. Before her were a set of pretty, white dishes banded in raised roses encircling the plates, cups, and saucers.

Dorothea fluttered and was pleased that I obviously liked the dishes.

"Do you entertain often?" she asked.

"I like having people over, but I'm not the cook that my mother was."

"Oh, how your mother could cook. Do you remember her pecan rolls, Lillian?"

"Oh, indeed. She was famous for her Sunday brunches."

Standing, I began to wrap and pack the dishes in the newspapers and boxes set aside for this task. Chatting away, I looked up from them and caught the view from their dining room window as the sun began to set in the sky.

I sat down. "How simply wonderful." I looked and looked. "Your view is breathtaking. You can really see the sun set perched on this lovely hill."

"Yes," said Lillian. "In all my travels, I have never enjoyed another view as much as this one. And Dorothea planted the hill as a park with paths to wander, walk, and sit beside."

Dorothea blushed from our praise. She'd planted their backyard hill in ferns, myrtle, birch, and four gnarled pines that shaded the landscape before us as the sky turned rosy, then gold before slipping into the earth below. Empty window boxes and urns once added patches of petunias, snapdragons, and sweet potato vines.

"You should see it when the tulips, daffodils, and hyacinths are up," said Lillian.

"Yes, but we can't stay, Lillian," said Dorothea, wringing her hands.

"Where are you going?" I asked.

"We're moving to assisted living," said Dorothea. "I'm so glad someone will have the white dishes who knows where their origin."

As we visited, they finished and filled in each other's words, such easy companionship. I learned about Lillian's deceased brother and how she had traveled last winter to the University of Iowa and stood to receive his distinguished alumni award for the one hundred patents registered in his name.

"We are the last of our line," said Lillian sitting ramrod straight. "Neither of us had any children."

I never even knew that Lillian had a brother. I only knew that Lillian, Dorothea, and Mabel were spinsters who thrived on attending University Women's Club and going to church. They had dinner parties and took trips together. I'd been in such a hurry to leave my hometown where I'd felt stifled as a hothouse flower as the middle school principal's daughter, that I ignored all the love that had surrounded me.

I took them to dinner to spend more time with them.

"If you see Mrs. Weber, please don't tell of our plans," said Lillian. "She's such a gossip."

"I won't tell a soul," I promised. "If anyone asks, I'll say that I've been given a gift by the ladies who still love and look after me." I added, "And I'll think of you and your house on Grand View Avenue whenever I use the white, rosebud dishes."

Driving home from Iowa, I was sorry that I hadn't put an offer on the Rockcliff house. It would be wonderful to have a home with such a view. The Monday upon my return, I biked up the Rockcliff hill. I couldn't believe my luck. The "for sale" sign still stood in the crabgrass yard of the double-decker house. That evening, I cajoled my husband into driving by it. He agreed to tour it the next evening. I had begun to imagine it cleaned up and downplayed the disarray.

Returning to our cozy brick bungalow after the realtor tour, my husband undressed, threw his clothes into the laundry chute, and disappeared into a hot shower. Emerging he asked, "What could you possibly see in that house?"

I shrugged and said nothing, understanding Andy's first view of the double-decker house. I knew my husband thought he was safe and the discussion closed.

The next morning before I went biking to the Borderline, I left Andy a list on the dining room table of what was right about the house.

<u>The Double-Decker House:</u>

Location, location, location.
The VIEW.
The two Florida Rooms stacked on the back for incredible valley views. The Jacuzzi tub in the downstairs unit. Ceiling fans throughout the house. Newly installed windows. Room for sons to visit. A rental retirement income if needed. A two car detached garage. A brick exterior. We could make money just fixing it up.
The view. The view. The view.
Location, location, location.

Two days later, we put a below tax value offer on the house. Three days afterwards, the owners agreed to sell to us, as other bidders had been disrespectful of their living conditions. For once, it paid off to be a social worker who had learned to have great tolerance for the living conditions of others. I was thrilled. Andy, who hated new expenses and *any* change, couldn't believe what we had gotten ourselves into. And, there was no going backwards because this time our cozy, brick bungalow sold in two weeks.

I wanted to slowly shape the house by cleaning and living upstairs first. Andy, on the other hand, was determined to move into a spotless house. He ripped up carpet. Scrubbed floors and walls. Painted. I kept quiet, uncertain who this whirlwind was and afraid of a tremendous rip in our relationship.

In the end, my husband gave his notice. "If you ever move again, you'll have to marry a younger man."

I kept quiet sorting through twenty-six years of family life in the brick bungalow. I knew better than to push my luck by complaining about all the work. Instead, my heart sang songs of homecoming while

Andy fretted that it would never be ready in time. Then he rounded up and hired our sons' available friends to get it all done on his time schedule.

Once we settled in, the double-decker house went beyond our expectations. Walking out the front door, we lived in the city. Walking out the back door, we were instantly in the country. Sitting on a bench at the edge of the cliff in our backyard, we watched the sun rise and set. The river sparkled below. The deer, rabbits, chipmunks, possums, raccoons, red-tail hawks, blue jays, long legged herons, and catbirds living in the emerald necklace woods below our bench entertained us endlessly. Joy bubbled within satisfying many hungers. The double-decker house would never let me forget this journey that has brought me to this extraordinary, living well, place.

"So we can see the sun rise at dawn."

Yes. We can. I had my house with a view and then some.

" Throw your dreams into space like a kite, and you do not know what it will bring back, a new life, a new friend, a new love, a new country."
—Anais Nin

Chapter Seventeen…Spring Rain

After moving into the double-decker house, everything seemed to be going my way. On the work front, the Ohio Attorney General began an audit of all the non-profit, foster care agencies in the state. Our *David* agency, which was the only one in our county and probably the only one statewide, told that we should be charging a dollar more for services rendered.

"It's so good to work for a small agency where every dollar counts and is spent on the kids." I sat across the desk from Bob, my new boss basking with him in the audit results.

"It's great to have your positive attitude and work ethic here," said Bob. "This is the first time I've cleared the paper off my desk in years."

During this honeymoon period, I settled in, planning to work at this agency for ten years or until I retired. The staff settled in also, and began to ask for my ideas on difficult situations. I was still carrying a 24/7 beeper, but what job was perfect?

On the home front, I continued to journal and shoot photos enlarging my vision during the first two hours of my morning before work. Carole (we shared not only the same name, but also a love of travel), Kim, and Sandy, whom I'd met at the Artist Way weekend, contacted me. Kim sent me an evaluation by the participants of my "point & shoot" workshop. There wasn't a negative one in the bunch and I was invited back for a repeat performance the next year. Sandy lined up two galleries that now carry my photo cards. Carole had a gift shop and wondered if I would put a big basket of cards there. A VP of a local college saw the cards and signed me on as a weekend contract photographer. And so it went. I set up a cottage industry in the second story sunroom. Perhaps, I was a real photographer after all. Life was good.

Prior to early morning biking, I'd agreed with many of my friends that spring skipped right through Cleveland in five minutes flat going from snow winter cold to summer humid hot. Clevelander's were just the recipients of hurricane trailers, the El Nino winds of the Panhandle Hook, and the notorious, "Lake Erie Effect." In my pre-diabetic, sedentary lifestyle, I rationalized that Cleveland's spectacular fall leaf show made up for a fragile, flowering spring of daffodils, azaleas, and tulip trees. One minute they were singing, the next they were either frosted cold or wilted hot never to flower again until next year. So it still surprised me when not a five-minute, but an eight-week spring, with all its seasonal splendor, springs itself on me while biking the metro park trails.

Accompanying spring was rain, torrents of it. On a recent morning, I'd lain in bed at three o'clock listening to the rain drumming its hands upon the land. I snuggled back into my bedcovers, resisting the temptation to click off my clock radio alarm, and fell happily back to sleep thankful that I was inside and dry. I dreamed of blue skies and sunshine.

At five, the radio announcer came on. "Twenty-nine degrees and falling. The rain will turn to snow showers this afternoon."

I clicked the voice off and listened to the rain, reluctant to move, debating my options. My husband was already up, puttering in the kitchen. Finally, I rolled out of bed, shrugged into my sweats, and dragged myself and my bike out into the unrelenting rain. My dad, who wintered in Arizona, always said it was easier to shovel rain rather than snow. I followed this axiom for the past three springs as a biking motto, but with poor results.

The Valley Parkway was dark, wet, and with water flowing everywhere in unexpected spillovers. Huge lake puddles covered sections of the all-purpose trail. I slithered through them slowly. These puddles were the texture of flour being stirred into a pan of bubbling water and beef drippings when making gravy. This standing water, getting colder by the minute, was thickening with dirt, twigs, and dead leaves.

When I arrived at the first bridge, the river was roaring. Its volume in noise matched its pulsating overflow. Tree limbs were being rushed to Lake Erie getting slammed and sometimes jammed into the curves of the banks. Why did all the picture books paint spring in fragile pastels?

It was a fantasy rather than a reality because most didn't experience spring except as a perfectly lovely day beckoning everyone outside like a Pied Piper. I could count on my fingers and still do the rare spring days of blissful beauty of tender greens under a clear sky, washed blue, with the temperature kissing the sixties. On the trails, spring was the hardest season of all to navigate despite the promise hinted at by Percy Bysshe Shelley saying, *If winter comes, can spring be far behind.* I needed to be careful for what I wished for in this life because things weren't always as they seemed. Right now, I was wishing for an umbrella.

Rain soaked through my winter white parka, seeping through my skin into the very marrow of my bones, chilling me cold. Winter had never treated me so rudely because the snow brushed aside easily. Ice was dangerous as I'd found out the hard way, but I'd stayed warm inside my protective parka and double-gloved hands throughout my bike hikes during winter. Previously, I had always thought of the rain as my friend, nourishing me as it had Alix Kates Shulman in her book, *Drinking The Rain.*

In her fifties, Alix Kates Shulman had gone to an island off the Maine coast to write in solitude and see what would become of herself without her usual audience. Would she disappear and become an "old biddy?" Finding abundance on her island, she began unbaggaging herself of wants promoted by the prevailing culture of her beloved New York City. She found, with the help of field guides on edible plants and sea creatures, an island treasure trove, free for the gathering of lamb's quarters, charlock flowers, mussels, and perwinkles. And, from the sky, she captured a clear water supply of rain in a cistern well. When she finally relaxed overcoming her "hacker" fears, Alix Kates Shulman became the Buddha saying, "You cannot travel on the path before you have become the path itself." She slowed her life for months to examine her interests and her future. Her transformational, midlife journey had not been kick-started with seven nights and six days in Vegas and then immersing herself right back into earning a living in a salaried position. *No, she'd probably be horrified to even contemplate such an outlandish idea.*

"Whatever for?" she'd ask me.

Although her message of island solitude inspired me and was just what the doctor ordered, the bigger problem with reading Alix Kates Schulman was that her densely woven storytelling made me feel inadequate as a writer. I was a fledging wren against her intricate words that reminded me of an oriole building a complex and strong nest.

The inner critic sitting on my shoulder kept saying, *This is how good writing reads.*

It took me days to answer back, *Yes, this is good writing if one is Alix Kates Schulman.*

And I took even longer to answer back. *But, even though I'm not an Alix Kates Schulman, it's okay. Get off my shoulder. Give me some room. My voice represents every woman who's envious of a Schulman and her months of solitude to sort herself out.*

My solitude was two hours every morning wrestled from my day to chew on while digesting the wooded, emerald necklace lessons of Cleveland. My voice, while not an oriole, reflected the busy wren population of humans.

I felt the belittler critic inside myself back off. I laughed at the Gods of Fate. I, too, was *"drinking the rain"* and I would write about my rain, which was not nourishing me at all.

Cold in the rain, I'd tried wrapping myself in a plastic garbage poncho. That helped but produced a sauna body bag complete with rivulets of sweat. Dehydrated after such rides, I drank glass after glass of tap water. Finally I broke down and went to *The Wilderness Shop* where nothing was cheap and free for the taking such as Schulman's mussels and charlock flowers.

"You need a rain jacket with vents," said a man half my age with a lean body. "The vents keep the body cool so that it won't get overheated. That's how pneumonia and other serious spring ailments get incubated."

My mother was probably applauding this decision to buy a rain jacket from her cloud seat in the heavens, telling my sedentary grandmother, "See. She knows the value of exercise. She takes after me. Don't you agree?"

I imagine my grandmother smiling back a Mona Lisa smile. She knew the real truth about her granddaughter.

I chose a hooded jacket that set me back ninety-five dollars. The double zipper worked from either top or bottom for good arm and leg action mobility or coverage depending on what was needed. Having a choice of either red or yellow, I decided I didn't want to be mistaken for an oversized park land duck. At last, I was dressed and protected from the windy torrents of spring. Trying the new jacket on in the privacy of a home mirror, I discovered that I would be venturing back into the forest disguised as Little Red Riding Hood.

What big puddles you are making, Mr. Rain.

All the better for bike riding. Think of it as melted ice.

And, I did, watching the parkway change. One by one, I saw the Hepatica, Bloodroot, Trout Lily, Dutchman's Breeches, Squirrel Corn, Blue Cohosh, White Trillium, and Blue Phlox creep over the land. These wildflowers popped up and sang with the chickadees, goldfinches, red-winged blackbirds and white-throated sparrows flying in from the south. The fish began their run upstream to lay their eggs. The great blue heron returned again, fishing in the open waters of the Rocky River. Scrawny deer crept down from the winter high grounds and feasted on the valley's spring's luncheon plate filled with greens and rain water. I could learn a lesson or two from the parkway about what to put on my plate.

When the budding canopy of tree leaves covered the land again, spring wildflowers said adieu to the sun and wouldn't flower again until next year. But for now, they flourished in the sun's spotlights and in turn, fed the first insects which fed the first amphibians and so on, as this continuous food chain supported the seasonal growth and wildlife of the Metro parks.

Summer would follow spring providing days of lengthy light and a land of plentiful nourishment. Nuts, apples, grapes, zucchini, sweet corn would be bountiful. No one would have to remind me to eat my vegetables fresh from the midwestern market stands.

Then the sun's rays would shorten as the earth turned its face. The green leaves would bow, change color, drop, and quilt the earth in red, yellow, brown, orange, and copper leaf patterns. The ground would blaze with vibrant colors. The sun's fading spotlight would usher in winter's entrance for Act IV. Then rain would turn to sleet, snow and ice stripping the ground carpet down to a dull brown while the forestland hibernated until spring arrived once again. Nature's plan had a purpose and gave me a sense of place, and a place to play in harmony with a map much larger than myself reminding me that change was a constant, the body was renewable, and some wishes did come true.

I remembered sitting in the Vegas library carrel dreaming of adding another book to my name. Maybe it was time to harvest my journals for essays about this midlife journey that I was on. Friends and colleagues noticed the weight loss and asked what I was doing.

"Biking," I answered. (I was still biking and watching my portions but I'd given up on Somersizing. It was too Un-American and so much more expensive. Restaurants didn't serve combination meals unless one ordered a la carte. Anyway, that's my excuse and I was sticking to it.)

"Why biking?" they asked.

"It's the only exercise I know how to do sitting down. It's a lazy woman's exercise." No wonder my grandmother was smiling down at me from heaven.

"But you can't bike in the winter, Carole."

I usually shrugged and changed the subject at this point in the conversation because if continued, it usually became argumentative in tone.

"So what's your favorite exercise?" I'd ask. Let them chew on that one for awhile.

However, I did decide to write an essay about biking year round. I entitled it, "The Boogeyman."

The Boogeyman: An Essay

When I pull myself out of bed at 5:30 a.m. and into my sweat suit, it is dark outside. December has arrived pushing the sun to the south. A wood of skeletons rattle their limbs as I ease my bike down Hogsback Lane into the Emerald Necklace Parkway that rings Cleveland, Ohio. Soon this season of winter, with masses of snow and ice, will complicate my morning exercise routine. I have found biking in the great out-of-doors unbelievably satisfying as it is a non-weight bearing activity that allows my fifty-year-old body to be a joyful kid again without the joint pains that many exercises cause me.

My husband is insistent about a bike light and mounts it himself despite being allergic to screwdrivers and product instructions. What I really need are night vision goggles as the bike light seems to illuminate me more than the street, which is fine as I don't want to end up as road kill. Every day now, I see either a dead raccoon, possum, or squirrel that hasn't made it across the road to the other side. My husband also wants me to add a referee's whistle to the bike key that I wear on a silver chain around my neck. I pooh-pooh this idea saying, "Silence is golden."

The truth is that one of the reasons I am so hooked on my morning bike rides is that it is blessedly quiet from the usual cacophony of human noise that besieges me daily as a social worker. In case I change my mind, the whistle rests in a dish on the kitchen window ledge.

Once comfortably on the park trail, I turn my bike light off as I like moving through the dark woods, my senses alert to the other animals getting up or going to bed for the day. I miss the soft light of summer, the damp mists of fall, but moving through the winter shades of night is also soothing. I am pedaling ten miles a day now. My drifting spirits soak in the solitude and are attuned to any unexpected rustles in the woods, or a panting runner, or a dog walker emerging out of the shadows on the trail ahead.

"It's winter and you're still riding?" My friends are in shock.

"You better believe it. Besides, we've hardly had any snow yet. I take my bike on a hike when the trails are slippery."

"What about the muggers and rapists?"

"They don't get up early."

"You aren't safe down there on your own."

"I'm in my second adolescence and feel invincible."

"Carole, be sensible. I have a cousin who was hurt when a rapist stuck a branch in her wheels, flipping her off her bike."

"What happened to her?"

"She managed to escape with the help of a jogger who heard her screams."

"I'm glad she had a loud voice and a guardian angel."

"Seriously, you should bike at the gym."

"Thanks for your concern, but part of the fun is being outside. If something happens, something happens. I refuse to live in fear and miss the other 364 days that the trails are friendly. I haven't felt so well in years."

And truthfully, my real fear is that I will stop and backslide into sedentary ways. Visions of amputated feet and blinding eye conditions propel me to treat exercise as a necessary prescription to being well. I want to use my feet and eyes while I have them. My blood sugar is dropping now rather than rising after cycling. (According to medical literature, this is an excellent sign that I'm getting my diabetes under control.) When I first started exercising, my blood sugars rose dramatically, and then eventually dropped a few hours later. My body has really been screwed up. Now my blood sugar is dropping by the time I finish my ride. So I promise myself that I will exercise every morning and if I miss a day, I'll continue the very next morning making it as routine as brushing my teeth. However, I do have to talk myself out of a cozy warm bed and don't need friends giving me excuses to quit.

Sometimes I waste a good twenty minutes fighting the darkness and resistance inside of me. I keep remembering the saying that resistance is the failure to accommodate necessary change. And my body needs this change because diabetes has set up camp permanently inside of me. My mantra becomes: "Bike for health. Everyday. Winter and diabetes will not defeat me because spring is just around the corner."

Once on the trails, my spirits soar. I revel in being outside, one with the texture of the day. Besides, the idea of floor-to-ceiling mirrors and lycra body suits at the gym just freak me out.

Such are my thoughts when I smell the cigarette smoke, which is unusual on the trails. Then I see him, a solitary smoker standing to the left of the trail leaning against a tree. This seems odd as the river is on the other side of the trail where most people stop while contemplating inner mysteries. I do not like the look of his loitering presence. I step up my pedaling passing him quickly hoping he isn't going to stick a tree branch in my wheels, flipping and flattening me to the ground. As I pass him, he turns his back hiding his face and the shape of his head in an upturned jacket collar. I roar on down the trail and do not slow my pace until I pass a pair of familiar joggers.

Why does this man trouble me so? As I slow my pace, I'm suddenly flooded with memories of fourteen-year-old me fleeing from a Y-Teen dance. I was not willing to spend the final hour at my first dance waiting for a ride home with Linda's parents. The man met on my flight home had also turned his back and hid his face in a turned-up collar.

The dance was a disaster on all counts. My hands were sweaty and I stepped on the foot of the only boy who asked me to dance. I was dressed wrong. The other girls wore matching sweater sets while I roasted in a hand knit, cable cardigan with a pretty pink blouse. The cardigan's bulk matched mine as I was changing into a girl with lots of curves. Sweater sets made my body look vulgar. The popular girls who were asked to dance were slim reeds of pre-pubescence. I fled the dance needing air and distance from my awkwardness. I took flight, walking along the night streets of my hometown of Clinton, Iowa, a sleepy river town on the banks of the Mississippi.

Just as I was feeling relieved and even enjoying my walk, I heard someone behind me. There were thirty-some, residential blocks ahead of me before I'd reach my front door, or I could retrace the eight blocks of deserted business streets that I had already covered and return to the dance. I picked up my pace while my follower was closing the gap between us. Just two weeks before, my father, a middle school principal, had warned me.

"Don't go wandering after dark by yourself." He sat at the dinner table having a second cup of coffee. "No need to alarm your friends, but it's important that you all stay together for safety. There is a rapist out there that the police are trying to catch."

I'd given anything to have remembered that admonition. My mind raced for an escape route. I could stop and phone my parents for a ride home at the Larson's house. My parents would be angry with me for leaving the dance alone, but I'd be safe.

Seven blocks later when I reached the Larson's on Third Street, their porch light was on, but my companion had disappeared. Not really wanting to explain why I wasn't at the dance to my parents, I continued on.

A block later he fell in behind me again. I was scared and then angry. I couldn't just wait to see what happened next. Walking briskly, I turned sideways and began speaking loudly to this man about the weather and the people I knew who lived along the street.

"Do you know the Larson's?"

Silence.

"Do you live near by?"

He mumbled something about friends and stumbled as if surprised by my conversation. He played with the zipper on his jacket. I worried about a knife as I walked sideways jabbering at him. As the county jail came into view, he turned off to see a friend.

I sighed with relief. But two blocks later, he was again behind me mumbling that his friends weren't home. I began chatting again. The tension between us was fierce. Not able to stand much more, I told him I lived on the next avenue, three houses down, the one with the roses.

"Have you ever noticed my mom's roses? She always says roses remind her of England, teacups, and biscuits. Isn't the white trellis pretty?"

I didn't live there but my grandmother and I often admired this house. As I turned off, my unwanted companion hesitated. I didn't.

"Thanks for the company."

He didn't say anything, but watched me skip down the side street and walk beneath the trellis with the climbing roses. Then I stepped into the shadows of the house. I crept gradually to the corner of the house and saw him still standing at the intersection, waiting. I froze. Mercifully, somewhere a door slammed.

He shrugged, turned around, and left. With my heart pounding, I waited in the shadows for an excruciating length of time. Had he really left?

I thanked God for giving me the courage to talk, the stamina to hide, and a slammed door. Finishing my prayer, I slipped into the alleyway behind the garages. I ran the next three blocks home reaching the safety of my back door.

My parents were playing cards with friends in the front living room. "Did you have fun?" asked my mom.

"It was okay."

"Do you have a boyfriend?" asked Mr. Reeves discarding a jack of hearts. "Were you kissed?"

"No," I said adamantly. My mother raised her eyebrows at me.

"Excuse me. I think I'll get ready for bed." I yawned. "I'm tired from all the dancing."

Once in my bedroom, I slipped under the covers fully clothed, cable knit sweater and all. I began shaking and crying softly while reliving my walk home. When my body finally quieted, I changed into a long-sleeved flannel nightgown vowing never to be so foolish again. I'd stay at a dance or not go at all. I certainly wouldn't wander off alone after dark.

Biking in the morning's darkness, however, feels different and is a most satisfying way to kick start a day. I know I'm vulnerable cycling in the Parkway, but I also know that there is tested courage inside of me to build upon. Besides, who would want to mug or rape an old lady?

As a social worker, I know the answer. Those that feed on evil, power, and control over others would.

The loiterer on the trail is now way behind me. The sun is starting to break night into day. My tires hum as I ride through the remaining woods and onto city streets again and into dawn's early light. I like the taste of freedom and it's worth managing the constricting fears of darkness to achieve it. The rapists and the muggers will not keep me from my morning bike rides. I don't have any magic wands to keep me safe, but I do know how and when to be noisy.

Even though I'm fiftysome now, I'll placate, soothe that gawky, fourteen-year-old girl inside of me so I can stay the course. Only then can I keep my focus and face the real boogeyman that is stalking my body, ready to pounce on my eyes, kidneys, and feet.

Once home, I retrieve the referee's whistle from the dish on the kitchen window ledge and add it to the silver key chain. I will keep my morning dance engagement with the woods.

"The fishermen know that the sea is dangerous and the storm terrible, but they have never found these dangers sufficient reason for remaining ashore."

—Vincent van Gogh

Chapter Eighteen... "Then I Saw Her"...An Opening

It was time for this writer to come out of hiding as the wildflowers do amongst the roots of the towering poplars, sycamores, and oak trees in the springtime. I'd test the literary waters at a writers' gathering of old friends and read aloud some vignettes about my disease. I rearranged my work schedule for their afternoon meeting, took a deep breath, and a dependable pen to write down their comments. I'd think about their reactions afterwards, when I was alone and could lick any wounds in private. It was smart to not be too defensive about reactions because then I wouldn't hear what was being said. Instead, I'd be like the Rocky River navigating myself around the sticks and rocks of my critics.

"Tone down the nature descriptions. Pure purple prose."

"What genre is this? Self-help, inspirational, memoir?"

"You have more than one story here. Which one is the real one? Is this going to be a book on diet & exercise, writing, diabetes, lifestyle changes?"

"How about a memoir of second chances?" I asked.

"It'll never get published," said Judy. "I'd center it around diabetes."

"Or, how about focusing on losing weight," said Alice. "That always sells."

Once they tore the themes and writing apart, the group quizzed me about my diabetes, weight loss, and bike riding. When did I discover that I had diabetes? Plus, the morning practices of journaling and biking intrigued them. What kind of bike was I using? How many days of the week did I really ride?

"Every day."

There was silence.

Finally, Alice said, "I don't believe you."

"I ride every day. I've done so for three years."

"You can't possibly ride every day," murmured Judy.

"Okay. I missed a day here or there due to an early morning work commitment or a few days when I had the flu last year. But, I rarely miss a day." I paused to let that sink in. "Otherwise, the routine of morning biking and writing practices wouldn't ever have been established. I'd spend too much time debating whether I could skip today. I resolved that issue when I realized that diabetes never takes a day off in my body."

I ran into Judy at the post office the next day. She stopped me to say how well I looked and how much my writing had touched her.

"You have to get published. I'll be the first in line to buy your book."

I glowed. Maybe it'd gone better than I thought.

"My husband was diagnosed with diabetes a year ago," she said. "I fear for him. He takes his pills but hasn't lost any weight or changed his habits."

I listened, empathized, and hopefully acted appropriate because concern for her husband loomed real over their lives. But inside, I was berating myself. Here, I'd thought she was complimenting me on my writing, not my weight loss.

Later I thought, maybe the two were not so separate. I'd touched her with my story, despite her disbelief that I couldn't possibly ride everyday and that the nature descriptions were overdone, bordering on purple prose.

I longed for a fellow writer to say, *I admire your work for the writing. You write like Emily Dickinson where every word counts.*

Instead, people honored what I had to say rather than how I said it. Maybe the story was the strength of the writing. Maybe the story couldn't be separated from the writing in good non-fiction. After all, I wasn't a poet like Emily.

To gain skills on sharing my journey, I enrolled in the Heights Writer's Conference. Driving there, I listened to *Wild Mind,* a taped reading by Natalie Goldberg on the censor in writing. She claimed that the censor made you write what you thought pleased others and made you sound like the All-American kid. Writing about a summer vacation, don't write, "I played baseball," when really you sat around polishing your toenails in all the colors of the rainbow or stayed in your room and out of the way because your dad had lost his job again.

Goldberg encouraged writers to read aloud with the *shaky voice* disease. "Let the writing out or it will fester. Hear what you are writing."

I agreed as long as my ego survived the reading and I could hear what touched the reader and what didn't.

Well-fortified, I was ready to face another writing audience, one that didn't know me. I never knew what to say and always ended up saying, *I played baseball on my summer vacation.*

I'd been drawn to the conference to hear Sherri Szeman, author of *The Kommandant's Mistress.* Sherri was sitting at the head table signing books. When I asked for her autograph, Sherri turned the proffered hardback over in her hands and asked how I'd come upon this first edition.

"When it was on the new arrivals table at my favorite bookstore, I was hooked with the first line, "Then I saw her.""

Sherri smiled.

Book signed, I found a seat and waited for the keynote pleased with myself. Sherri Szeman began with humor, listing as non-believers, even her family who found any desire to write strange. Sherri was teaching full-time at an Ohio college when she wrote her first novel following all the rules. However, she couldn't find a publisher. Discouraged, she asked the English Department chairperson if she could have a one-year sabbatical without losing her tenure. She was told that she could have her tenure, but not her salary. Before she changed her mind, Sherri went to the bank and asked for a loan to write a novel. After much consultation, Sherri was given an $18,000 loan to write her second novel with 18% interest attached. She would begin her loan repayment nine months from the date of the loan.

No wonder Sherri's family thought writing made her crazy. I could just hear Andy's reaction to the idea of taking out a loan to write a book.

Sherri cried all the way to her apartment fearful of what she had done. Once home, she dried her tears and set to work. She didn't follow the rules this time, conceiving and writing out of herself, *The Kommandant's Mistress.* This was *her* money and she would write to please herself.

Shades of my diabetic journey jumped out at me as I listened. I cheered Sherri on, remembering the counseling truism, *Don't try, try, try the same old thing again. Try something different.*

Sherri wrote Kommandant Maximilan von Walther's part first. Then she discovered who and how poet Rachel Sarah Levi reacted and acted in sharing the same history and space as his enslaved mistress. The book's stark words drew the reader into the power struggle between these two voices and their final meeting.

Sherri had written a story that I couldn't put down, and I longed to be so talented.

Later sitting in Sherri's afternoon workshop, she identified her use of man versus man as the conflict used in her opening line, "Then I saw her." Next, she called on me as the lady in the lavender sweater. *No, I hadn't worn an authoritarian, career outfit. I'd worn a lavender turtleneck with my Vegas blue jeans.*

"Give me another universal conflict."

The writers around me saw my startled reaction and whispered an answer so I wouldn't have to say that *I didn't know, because I played baseball on my summer vacation.*

"Man versus God," I stammered.

"Good," said Sherri. "That's The Book of Job."

The workshop continued to roll. We were given writing exercises and I found myself focusing on how to begin my journey with urgency and conflict. I knew through my journaling that the real conflict was not daughter vs. mom, woman vs. nature, nor woman vs. God, but rather woman versus her *buried* self.

Sherri circulated the room as pens moved across paper. She read my first five lines out loud, and then said, "I would read more of this."

Sherri Szeman liked my beginning words. I glowed. I did handstands in my seat.

I'd live on that praise for a long time nudging the writer from within to come out of hiding, fighting for words to tell my story. I couldn't take in the last workshop of the afternoon because my mind was too full and singing with relief. *I am a writer who can write more than parenting books.*

I drifted instead into the ballroom. I helped myself to a cup of freshly-made coffee while snubbing the chocolate cake. *Who needs chocolate cake? I was already feeling joyful.*

I sat at an empty table filling out an evaluation and sipping coffee when Sherri Szeman came in, looked around, and joined me.

"You have a story to tell, Carole. My hope for you is to keep writing it."

I'd been given permission to write more by an author I respected. *Thank you, Sherri Szeman.*

And thank you, Natalie Goldberg. Thank you, Emily Dickinson. By sharing your voices, the way opened before me. Knowing guidance was there by diligently searching for answers, I'd continue. I'd bike through the parkway disguised as Little Red Riding Hood gathering stories, ready to overcome any critical wolves, especially the censor from within.

What big ears you have.

All the better to hear you with my dear.

And I would be heard and I'd hear others as they taught me the way. *And thank you, ladies of the afternoon writers' club. I will remember what you heard, liked, and I'd build on those themes. I'll weed out the purple prose, but not the Valley Parkway and its biking trails.*

And thank you, Bob, for hiring me. I was establishing a writing routine without battling the chaos of a sixty-hour work week. I really was only working forty-hours a week.

On the right path, I'd bloom while biking and writing through the metroparks, at the Borderline, and beyond. The lines begun in Sherri's workshop highlighted the conflict of woman vs. self. Whether I used them or not didn't matter. What mattered was that I'd given myself an opening—a second chance to not only examine my outlook on life, but to move past the *shaky voice* syndrome. The words wouldn't fester inside, as I'd hear them and identify what I was feeling. I had diabetes, which had sparked a new writing journey. I'd write about how it all began. After all, Sherri Szeman liked my opening lines.

Blurred Vision: An Essay

I took my foot off the accelerator and safely snaked my blue Buick Regal into the slower right lane on Cleveland's inner belt. Beads of sweat had popped out all over my body. To keep my hands from shaking, I gripped the steering wheel as I strained to make out the white letters on the green highway signs, the letters blurring into a sea of murky glop. What was wrong with me?

Thirsty, I swallowed to unstick my tongue from the roof of my mouth. This had to be more than the latest office virus. Much more.

As the director of a case management agency, I'd pushed myself to honor a work appointment because this meeting had taken six weeks to set up. I didn't want to reschedule it and wait another six. The contract needed signing if we were to get paid in a timely fashion at this year's rate.

All through the early afternoon meeting, I'd promised myself I would go straight home as soon as it was over. No more office work for me today. With an upset tummy, I'd sit in the family room recliner, drink icy ginger ale, munch on saltine crackers, and take my first sick time in seven years.

Meeting successfully over, I decided that there was no way that I was going home now that my vision had blurred accompanied by white, confetti sparks. The fear of going blind had haunted me since childhood with each new corrective layer that was added to my thickening spectacles. When I finally stopped growing at age thirteen, my eyes stabilized and by age fourteen, the doctor didn't need to adjust my lenses anymore.

"I can still see," I announced, my body flooding with relief. "I'm not going to be blind."

"Of course not," said the eye doctor. "Your eyes just changed as you grew tall. You were never in any danger of going blind. I told you that."

(I had never believed that explanation, thinking the adults were humoring me, not wanting to frighten me about my inevitable fate. I had thought that it was only a matter of time until I joined Helen, my friend from church, at the School for the Blind.)

A year later, I was fitted for contacts and hid my near-sighted eyeglasses beside my locked diary in my underwear drawer.

Now what was wrong with my eyes? At age fifty, I did have glaucoma, but this was beyond the creeping vision losses that defined that condition. Once I recognized my exit by landmarks, I drove directly to the ophthalmologist's office determined to sit in his waiting room until he could see me.

"You did the right thing," said Dr. Bennett, my eye doctor for twenty years. "I'm glad you came straight here."

His assistant darkened the room. A bright light was shone into my eyes while I obeyed his commands. "Look up. Look left. Now down. Now to the right. Again. Look up. Now left. Down. To the right."

Next he checked my eye pressure putting the cold, black metal, facemask machine with swinging, miniature probe torches against my eyes.

I unstuck my tongue from the roof of my mouth and whispered hoarsely, "Is it macular degeneration?" Macular degeneration, a blinding eye condition, runs in the family.

"No."

"A detached retina?'

"No."

"Why is everything blurry? Why can't I focus? What do I have?"

"Your eye pressure is a little elevated, but normal, and your central vision is intact." He paused. "Tell me, Carole, what have you been eating?"

Eating? What did food have to do with going blind? All my life food had defined me one way or another. My mother, my grandmother, my dad, and my brother were suddenly sitting in the examining room with me.

"Have another biscuit," urged my stout grandmother proudly passing her homemade contribution to Sunday dinner.

My petite mother frowned as she passed grandmother's legendary biscuits without taking a second one. Dad slipped another on his plate. My brother, John passed, saying that he was full while rubbing his stomach in contentment. My mother beamed at him, then gave a frown to grandmother as I gingerly placed another biscuit on my plate looking forward to slathering it with butter and mom's strawberry jam. This urging to take a second biscuit and the frowns passed between the matriarchs in the family happened at every Sunday dinner of my childhood.

"What does eating have to do with my eyes?"

"Just answer the question, Carole."

"Well," I hedged. "I haven't been feeling well."

"Go on."

"I haven't really been eating because I must have the flu and that's why I can't keep anything in me. I've been nibbling on applesauce, Jell-O, saltine crackers, ice cream, and sipping ginger ale."

"Why aren't you home in bed?"

"I was going there, when everything went blurry, with shooting lights."

"I think you have adult onset diabetes."

Diabetes!

"Your vision will clear up when you are feeling better. In the meantime, avoid sugary foods and make an appointment with your internist right away. And, I'll want to see you in two weeks to recheck your eye pressure. Any questions?"

"No," I said unable to think while my mind kept shouting the diagnosis.

Diabetes! No way. I had the office virus. I couldn't have diabetes. It didn't run in the family.

Driving slowly home, diabetes and its warning signs read long ago in a magazine article flitted around the periphery of my vision. I did have glaucoma, which can be a warning sign that diabetes might be waiting in the wings. I'd also given birth to a ten-pound, baby boy on my last trip to the delivery room, another sign. I was also an *apple* rather than a *pear* shaped matron whom carried her weight in her abdomen rather than her hips.

Arriving home, I phoned my internist's secretary, heated some milk, and poured it over a slice of dry toast in a soup bowl. I choked down this penance meal of milk toast, the food I dreaded and was spoon-fed when I was sick as a child. (As a result, I wasn't sick much as a child.) When my husband arrived home, I said I wasn't feeling well and put myself to bed.

The next morning, I could see perfectly. The sparks and the blurred edges were gone. I swore off Jell-O, applesauce and ginger ale, but hedged on the ice cream. I'd eat less of it and eliminate the hot fudge topping. In fact, I threw the jar of hot fudge in the trash, bagged it, and buried it in the ten-gallon garbage can outside.

Two days later, I kept my appointment with my internist, humoring the eye doctor's fears. Plus, I couldn't go back for another pressure check and say that I'd ignored his suspected diagnosis.

"I'm fine. Really. I just had the office virus, but Dr. Bennett insisted that I see you."

To be safe, my internist sent me to the lab to have blood drawn. Then I went on about my business working the usual sixty-hour week. *Who has time to get preoccupied by fleeting symptoms, even blinding ones? This had been a fluke incident, hadn't it?*

Two weeks later, my internist sent me a letter unable to reach me at home and hesitant to leave an unauthorized message with my husband.

"I have tried to reach you by phone multiple times. Your serum glucose is very significantly elevated to 377 mg/dl. Although you may need insulin, I would like to place you on *Diabeta* immediately; 5 mg. in the morning, 5 mg. at supper, and ask you to follow up with me in 10 days. It is extremely important that you follow up and I look forward to hearing from you."

DIABETES! I CAN'T HAVE DIABETES!

How had I come down with this disease?

Deep inside I knew why, because eating with abandon had caught up with me at last. I'd now pay for all those second biscuits and other helpings of delectable food that I loved. I didn't know restraint, never had when it came to food.

Guilty as charged. Shame on me.

Ten days later, I sat in my internist's office and was told that I had Type 2 Diabetes, and that it could be controlled through diet, exercise, and pills. Losing fifty pounds would also help as fat decreases the body's efficient use of insulin.

"A pound a week ought to do it," said my doctor. "A year from now, we'll see where you are and if you need insulin."

Losing weight was a tall order. I wasn't at my current weight because I hadn't tried dieting. I hated dieting because it made me dizzy, shaky, and sick. Pounding headaches were a sure accompaniment.

Plus, whom was she kidding? I didn't need to lose 50 pounds. Seventy pounds was more like it!

A pound of flesh a week. I would pay dearly for the sin of gluttony.

"I began to write short pieces when I was living in a room too small to write a novel in."
—Angela Cartwright

Chapter Nineteen...Second Story Woman

When we moved to our double decker abode, my husband wanted to live down and I wanted to live up. This disagreement resolved itself when we agreed to not have a tenant until we got both units in order. We'd live up and down for nine months while we fussed over our *must do* list: install whole house air-conditioning, lay linoleum in the sun rooms, build a usable bathroom in the basement, renovate the basement office for me, erect a slatted patio roof over the back deck, install a gas grill, and level and landscape the back yard.

The blue sky, clouds, and seagull stained glass frame was too big for the window seat nook in the first floor living room, so it was hung upstairs for a northern view. The upstairs living room gradually evolved into a temporary family room. Mounted photo groupings were hung on the ample wall space turning the upstairs into Carole's personal art gallery.

The upstairs master bedroom was painted a blue haze that turned purple in a certain light. White shutters and a white, oversized curlicue mirror accented this room's clean peacefulness. Mary's writing table was placed under the window framed in white eyelet.

In the smaller upstairs bedroom that was connected at the hip to the Florida sunroom, I set up a temporary office. Two computers, two printers, a fax machine, file cabinets, halogen light, bulletin boards, and book cases. Books overflowed into the Florida room with its floor to ceiling bookshelves. Wonderful books on photography, nature, memoir, and mysteries surrounded me.

There, a round table with cushioned wicker chairs joined them, as did a bamboo chaise lounge rescued from the trash pile with quilt thrown over its tattered, plumb pillows. This became a sunny reflective room with a view of the valley that was incredible from the upper deck of the house. I smiled thinking of my grandmother, Dorthea, and Lillian and their rooms with a view. I had joined them at last. My grandmother always said, "If you have a view, the world will come to you." My mother's quote also fit this *soul-soaring* sunroom. "If you can read, you can do anything." The matriarchs in my life came into accord at last. I took up complete residence in the upper unit.

I made photo cards from my best valley shots to announce our new residence sitting at the round table while surveying the Rocky River below me. Next came the creation of dried flower pictures along with favorite sayings decorated with yard flowers of Johnny jump-ups, fuschia, geranium, and verbena. The light, view, and space encouraged my creative passions. Plus, my early morning writing sessions in my home office in the sky allowed Andy to sleep soundly downstairs. When I'd crept out of bed in the middle of the night in our former ranch home, he got up cranky saying that I'd kept him awake with my wanderings.

Andy set up the downstairs kitchen. No longer hampered by a tiny, ranch-style, galley kitchen, he set up shop blissfully making muffins, slow cooker dishes, and grilling on the back deck. Friends came over, feasted, and marveled at our view. We began taking a lot of kidding. "Does Andy have visiting privileges upstairs, Carole?"

"Sometimes," I quipped.

Others confided in my husband, "I think you've found the secret for a happily married life."

Michael, our first-born, came for a visit and stayed in the upstairs unit. "It's perfect. You have a big kitchen, Dad," he chuckled. "And, Mom has a studio."

"A studio." That lovely phrase caught, stuck, and focused my mind. "A studio." I had never thought of the upper unit that way.

"Well, she better not get used to it because we're moving her office to the basement and renting out the upstairs."

I didn't say a word and our son's eyes locked onto mine.

"It will take dynamite to get Mom downstairs, Dad."

I now knew what Mona Lisa was smiling about. I also knew now was not the time to discuss tenants when we already had an agreement to live in the whole house for nine months and only three months had passed. I changed the subject to our son's new job. But my husband couldn't leave the studio label alone after our son left.

"Two people don't need this much space."

"Says who?"

"We are in the down-sizing era."

"Why? We're still growing, changing."

"Think of all the people who don't have enough room."

"Does that mean I can't create my own space and not feel guilty about it?"

"If we don't rent the top unit, this house will never get paid off."

"So? I like living in the sheer pleasure of the moment for now."

"You're usually more practical, Carole."

"How about we rent out the first floor unit?" I asked

"No way. It has more living space with the deck and yard."

"I like living with light and my art."

"You'll like the basement office when its finished. We'll put lots of lights in it."

"It doesn't have a view."

And so it went.

Writer, Natalie Goldberg, discussed this space issue about women artists in her book, *Living Color*. Natalie said she had made "a religion of writing in cafes—not having my own studio, making it egalitarian...Was I afraid of occupying my own dimensions, of actually pushing out walls for myself?" As a social worker, I had similar thoughts about egalitarian living. But I, too, began to examine my feelings of pushing out walls for myself.

Apparently many artists, particularly women artists, didn't have separate studio space. Like women everywhere, they made their rooms serve overlapping functions: the kitchen table became the writing table, a den was also the guest room, the laundry room might sport an easel or computer table, the basement half bath doubled as a dark room, a cutting table was set up in the middle of the living room to lay out fabric or worksheets for an artist's space station. I realized that it was pure luxury to walk into studio space ready to begin or resume any project, undisturbed. But, it was fast becoming a necessity for my well-being. It may take dynamite to get me out of the upstairs studio space. Or, bankruptcy. Or, death.

When I went to Iowa to pick up the *white dishes*, I'd not only visited Dorthea and Lillian, but also revisited the home of my childhood. The current owner still painted it gray with white trim, but had enclosed the screened front porch into a year-round room. They'd miss the summer breeze caressing the face, sipping black cow sodas in the glider, and neighborly chatter on the porch. The scent of bridal bushes wouldn't perfume the air below screened windows as they had been removed and decorative flower boxes had been added. The shutters my mom and dad had rescued, then sawed, and fit into the living and dining room windows were still in place. I didn't ring the bell asking for a peek inside. I knew I wouldn't find my mom's legendary brunch spread out in the dining room or the Winslow painting of the sea hanging in a gold frame over the couch.

Instead of knocking on the door asking for a house tour, I took a few photos to view later as the house on Third Street that Carole grew up in. Mom and Dad would have been pleased at how well the house looked. Someone new was raising kids here as a tricycle was parked in the back yard under the maple tree that I had loved to climb. It was as big as I remembered having grown in my memory banks to its current size. *It would never be too big for its britches like I'd grown.* Well, I was working on that. I said hello and goodbye to my old friend.

Walking the back alley and around the block, I recognized landmarks but I didn't recognize any of the folks that I passed. I knew no one and no one knew grown-up me in the old neighborhood. The principal's daughter had escaped at last. This small town not only knew most everyone, but most everyone had an opinion of me. *Does she get straight A's because she's smart, or because of whom her father is? It's too bad, Bookworm, that your brother got the long eyelashes and the good looks. Tsk. Tsk. Did you see Carole holding hands and kissing, walking along the river? What's she doing, going out with a college boy, anyhow? She's only in high school. If he can't control his daughter, he's in no position to be giving out detentions to our children.* It felt good to have outgrown all that childhood angst. Growing up here, I'd never recognized myself outside of this small town's scrutiny. Escaping to a big university had been such a relief.

After revisiting my childhood haunts, I went to the cemetery where my mom was buried. As it was the weekend, there was no one in the Lawn Cemetery's office to ask where my mother's ashes were interred. I walked the rows while a red brown dust covered my sandals and sifted through to paint my feet with grave dust. But, I couldn't find Mom. I'd sleep on it and would try again tomorrow morning before leaving town.

I next went to where Grandmother Thuresson was buried. My grandmother had been disappointed when mom and dad had not bought the gravesite next to the Thuresson plot. My grandmother liked a gravesite with hills, stories, and statues, while my mother like memorial cemeteries with plain white markers. Their final resting-places matched their personas. Both were gone now but they still visit me in dreams with conflicting tales and ideas.

Grandmother was buried in Rose Hill Cemetery down a country road that I remembered as if I'd traveled it only yesterday. I'd visited this gravesite frequently as a child as my grandmother liked to call on grandfather after Sunday dinner. She liked to sit awhile under the shade of a white pine in a canvas chair while she directed me to weed, deadhead petunias and snapdragons, and to fetch water from a ground spout up the hill by the custodian's shed.

Everything was as I remembered it. I couldn't believe that nothing had changed. Even the memorial for the Tornado of June 3, 1860 still stood surrounded by the white tires. The marker read that 20 persons were killed and buried in this plot. It went on to say that "228 homes, churches, school, hotels, warehouses, stables and businesses" were destroyed. A cali lily was etched into this granite marker looking for all the world like a white tornado. The victims were nameless and I wondered if their families ever knew what had happened to them? And were the rubber tires to protect them in death from another tornado touchdown? As an adult, I still found this gravesite disturbing.

One minute you're here. The next, you aren't. Scary thought. Better get busy living was the message I focused on.

Grandmother's grave looked robust and the white pine continuously decorated the Thuresson plot with petite pinecones. I read the headstones once again. Baby Leonard Lee was buried here, as was his father, my grandmother's third son, Ralph. Divorced, Uncle Ralph's wife was buried somewhere else. But father and baby rested at my grandparents' side. Grandfather had lived only 65 years while grandmother had lived on for sixteen more years to age eighty-one.

I sat down, incredulous. Eighty-one years! Why, my grandmother, who'd eaten herself into a heart attack according to my mother, had lived longer than I thought. How could that be? My athletic mother starved to death in the vise of Lou Gehing's disease and died at age, seventy-eight. What did this mean for my future? Didn't eating right matter after all? Wouldn't you know that my mind would go to food, even at a cemetery? Of course it mattered what I ate. I had diabetes.

I continued to sit and visit for awhile. I thanked Grandmother for her sense of color and pattern. Her quilts made my home a warm place for the eye. I liked looking at her art. I thanked her for the fairy tales, myths, and Bible stories that we had read out loud, ensconced and surrounded by the light streaming through turret windows. I also thanked her for her stubbornness in insisting on being a second story woman surrounded by friends. Finally, I thanked her for being my Grandmother and loving me.

As I said good-bye, I left a smiling faced, clay head on her rose granite marker that Michael, her first great grandson of her only daughter's daughter had made when he was in kindergarten. I thought she would like this face and remembrance of family on her headstone. Then I picked some pinecones off her grave to take with me to place in a blue bowl at home on the Clausen half table that Grandfather had rescued from a fire. My family shrine remains, reminding me of life's possibilities.

Early the next morning, I stopped again at the Lawn Cemetery with a bouquet of fresh flowers. As a child I had begged to come to this cemetery because a pond with a pagoda, blue spruces, and weeping willows had been created near the entrance. Two pure white swans with eyes masked in black still swam there. I'd always marveled at their long necked, Audrey Hepburn bodies. I could only dream to be as graceful as they were in gliding across the water. I'd never tired of watching them or remembering the story of the hopeful story of the "ugly duckling" sitting on a stone bench.

I went to this stone bench and again watched the swans. *Where was Mom buried?* I remembered her saying that she and dad had purchased a plot next to the Lincoln Highway. I walked through the Whispering Pines section near the highway but couldn't find her. I looked particularly close at graves with no plastic flowers. A standard was provided for a simple flower offering. Mom would have hated all the silk and plastic flowers as she had liked this cemetery for its clean lines and grassy plots.

Next, I tried the Rose Garden section and found her at last. She lay exposed to the Iowa sky with a clear road to heaven. The dates on her headstone proclaimed her seventy-eight years of life. Life certainly has no set timetables. It was best to live in the now, full out. I put a crescent stone in the urn crease to say I'd visited and I laid the fresh flowers on her grave. I knew they would be withered by the end of the day, but they were as real as she had once been.

I bowed to her from the waist and thanked her for my life. I told her that I was trying to lose my stubbornness about eating for comfort and pure pleasure. I thanked her for the discipline and strength that she had shown and taught me by example throughout her life. She felt cheated when dying of Lou Gehrig's disease; she who had always taken such good care of her body. She wasted away and labored for every breath as her carbon monoxide levels overtook her swimmer's deep lung endurance. Her doctors couldn't believe that she was still alive and offered her relief in the form of a respirator. She pushed the suggestion aside. The cells in her brain were not going to regenerate and send the signals to tell her muscles to move. These muscles had withered and died one by one as mom lost the ability to swallow and to eventually breathe in oxygen and expel the carbon monoxide. Having read about her disease, she knew what she knew, and died unaided by machines.

The nurse who attended to her after her death said Mom looked so peaceful. She said, "Dying well means one has had a good life."

I thanked the nurse for her kind words. My mother had truly been a long distance swimmer and faced her death with presence.

"Love you, Mom."

I went and sat by the swans for awhile being soothed by their grace. Beauty surrounded me as I glided across the pond with them. I took a few swan photos in this garden of reflection. When finished, I stumbled on a stone at my feet. Within the fossilized holes, I saw a face there, a familiar face. I put the stone in my bag to carry with me as I left this resting-place ready to resume my life's journey.

When we settled into the double decker house, I took mother's stone out of my camera bag and put it in my sunroom to grace me with her presence. Michael had intuitively understood about the sacred space that I had created proclaiming, "Mom has a studio." I saw empty space and put it to wonderful use. Rainer Maria Rilke writes: "We are not to fear the strangeness we feel. The future enters into us long before it happens."

Sitting in the Garden of the Enigma, I'd wondered if I was old or young, a visionary, or a dreamer. I didn't need to choose, for I was all. Who knew that I'd stop being a busy bee and look within to create art that pleased me?

Nine months have now passed since we came to live well in the double decker, Rockcliff House. There are no more discussions of tenants. Even Andy isn't protesting anymore about using too much space. He has the downstairs kitchen uninterrupted to play full out at being a chef. In the morning, Andy sits in the first floor sunroom reading his paper, listening to his tunes, and then strolling with his coffee mug to the picnic table at the end of the yard overlooking the river. With his aviator eyesight, Andy watches hawks, herons and wood finches. I can see him from my studio getting myself dressed and ready to ride to the Borderline Café.

My husband and I have come full circle. The nest was empty of children and parents who currently are on their own journeys. The pair of us remained intact, happier than ever. In this house, solitude and companionship were both possible. In this house, anything seemed possible—even a studio of one's own with a towering view. I couldn't miss what I didn't have and I've fallen in love with studio space and the husband and family that supports me there. I never wanted to work a sixty-hour week again. I liked being a social worker and an artist passionate about living well. I have biked way beyond the borderline of my old life bringing the best of my many-sided selves to reside in the best double decker of them all. I was home. I was a second story woman.

"Something we were withholding made us weak
Until we found it was ourselves."
—Robert Frost

Chapter Twenty...In My Husband's Kitchen

I was impatient to get to the Borderline and to my journal writing. Words had been flying unchecked across the page yesterday, when four words jolted me into a new awareness. These words were, *In my husband's kitchen.*

Entering the Parkway, I pulled my red hood over my biking helmet before negotiating Hogsback Hill and the unchecked wind that was whipping through naked trees. My eyes teared peering out behind my glasses on the lookout for patches of slick leaves. The shrouds of this week's work tensions vanished by the time I reached the bottom of the hill and began soaking in the Parkway's solitude and stark beauty. It was a Friday with lots of work behind me and what lay ahead would be all downhill giving me freedom this weekend to ride the Emerald Necklace's trails at length with my camera and notebook. A squirrel startled me by scampering across my path reminding me to look, listen, and breathe deeply while in the Valley Parkway. I took a few cleansing breaths letting the oxygen reach the tips of my toes. Tilting my head way back, I marveled at the tree arms stretching so tall, reaching forever upwards despite a good shaking by the wind. Then I tore down the trail on my bike, riding out of pure joy and becoming one with the wind, trees, and the pathway.

My mind flitted around the phrase, *in my husband's kitchen.* The fact of this truth reverberated throughout my body as I pumped the tires round and round. Before I knew it, I was halfway up the Detroit Hill and was still going strong. Breathing hard now, I made it to the top without stopping once.

I did it! I rode all the way up the Detroit Hill and out of the Valley Parkway.

At the top, I dismounted and hugged myself in astonishment while breathing deeply to slow my rapid heart beat. Looking down the hill, I could barely see the bottom. My biking had strengthened my limbs like a woodland tree forever reaching skyward.

Kelly greeted me with coffee at the Borderline. I ordered oatmeal with blueberries and cinnamon. We rejoiced in the victory of biking up and out of the Valley Parkway, both impressed with such a performance. Then I settled down to write.

I titled the page, *In My Husband's Kitchen.* The kitchen in our Rockcliff home fitted Andy like a wrap-around apron. I usually sat waiting for dinner at the built-in table as an audience of one while my husband cooked all around me.

My husband would be happy in his second life by being a short-order cook. Andy cajoled any company, including repairmen, with food. Homemade muffins, rice puddings, pasta salads, farm omelets, pierogies and onions, root stews, and cabbage stir-fries were readily available in his kitchen. The children and I understood that no one entered the chef's territory when he was in it. As a temperamental cook, Andy kept everyone, including me, effectively out of *his* kitchen. I'd been happy to do so and had always thought that this was a good deal. But was it?

When my husband and I originally divided up household chores, I suspected Andy failed laundry on purpose, unless one likes colorful underwear. That left food shopping, which eventually led him to being the main cook, a role he delighted in performing. I'd been glad that my husband encouraged my career and didn't expect me to do it all. But, then, smart man that he was, Andy didn't have to do it all either.

However, there was another reason I probably stepped so willingly aside in the kitchen. In my childhood home, I'd been taught to step aside. That kitchen was mom's. I was in it only if eating, drying the dishes, or decorating holiday cookies. My mother didn't have a short fuse like my husband. Instead she had *the look* that didn't brook any interference or encroachment of her supplies.

Food and meal management were Mom's territory. Once she put her apron on, she was all business. My mom was an outstanding cook. I didn't know anyone of her acquaintance who'd have preferred eating at any restaurant compared to dining at her table. But the bottom line for me was that I felt awkward in my mother's kitchen and at her meals. There everything was regimented and in its place. A sugar bowl never graced her table as they did at friends' homes to sweeten cereal, tea, and even grapefruit. When it came to food, I was brought up as a purist, unsweetened.

Alone, in the kitchen of my first apartment, I learned to cook and bake by trial and error. I had a good sense of how to pull a meal together having watched mom's performance from the sidelines. And to give me an edge, I exchanged a new *Betty Crocker Cookbook* for my mom's well-thumbed copy with the recipes for snickerdoodle cookies and vegetable barley soup. Mom had always said that if you could read, you could learn how to cook. So I became a good cook in the family tradition of fine cooks. I even discovered dishes that mom pronounced excellent and copied such as my scalloped oyster dish, baked chicken stuffed with crab, bran muffins, and *Popeye* meatballs. With Mom's official seal of approval, I'd arrived as a first class cook.

However, since my husband had commandeered the kitchen, my bookshelves bulged with cookbooks that I'd long since abandoned. I no longer consulted them except on special occasions to check what temperature to roast the holiday turkey or to check the flour and milk measurements for making Yorkshire Pudding. But when I did, I'd find myself reading them and thinking that I'd like trying some new dishes. But I never took the time to do so.

Why had I stopped reading and trying out recipes for pure entertainment? When had I given up cooking? Why had I given the kitchen completely to my husband? Had I really lost interest in preparing food? Or, was it that I never really thrived in the kitchen? It certainly didn't fit me like a glove as it did my husband.

When we started a family, I remember taking a vow that *my* children would never belong to the Clean Plate Club. Wanting my children to be more relaxed about eating than I was, I went overboard in the opposite direction.

"Eat. Don't eat. I don't care."

But I did care. Food was being wasted and the children were hungry when I was in the middle of doing something else. I created mealtime monsters and needed to find a middle ground. I gave them a new message.

"Eat something, because I'm not cooking until the next meal. There's peanut butter and jelly for sandwiches if you don't like what's on the table."

Mealtimes became more relaxed. Then I stopped putting together a complete dinner of an entree and with three side dishes of vegetables and salads. The kids didn't want big meals but Andy complained that he liked a complete meal with a couple of side dishes. Sometimes I'd stick an onion or a loaf of thawed bread dough in the oven to perfume the house. That stopped his complaints. It at least smelled like someone was cooking in the kitchen. *There's those aromatic molecules, volatiles, at work for Andy, and for me.*

I'd long marveled at my neighbor's attitude towards food and her children. In her opinion, planning three meals a day was a waste of time. Instead, breakfast and lunch were on your own at her house. Cereal, toast, cheese, fruit, crackers, and canned soups were always available when anyone felt like eating. A delivered pepperoni pizza was often dinner. When she did get around to cooking, everyone welcomed the meal. Everyone was slim at her house. This relaxed attitude toward food was a message I needed to learn because I was fat and diabetic.

Neither my husband nor I belonged to the Slim People's Club. Meals were so important in our respective childhood homes that our mothers knew what the next meal would be before we'd finished the one we were eating. Mom had the final say, so I never got too excited about such discussions which often continued while doing the dishes. So I talked about other things while I dried the silverware and she polished the bottoms of her pans.

Working on a different kitchen atmosphere, I invited the children into the kitchen to stir the gravy, time the spaghetti, season the soup, or toss a salad. We cooked meals together. Family cooking destroyed my wedding set of pots and pans. As I replaced them, my mother looked on in disapproval. She had one set of pots and pans throughout her entire adult life and while worn, they were still perfect with copper, bright bottoms. I knew Mom thought I was careless and didn't know how to look after things. But, I was looking after other things.

She had been amazed when Andy took over the kitchen becoming a short-order cook for our sons. She'd have been fully amazed when my dad taught himself to cook more than scrambled eggs and toast after her death, and began exchanging recipes with Andy.

Our children are now grown, Mom was no longer in the kitchen except in my head, and I'd let our kitchen become my husband's domain. Perhaps part of my attraction to fast foods wasn't a reward for working, but was an avoidance of the kitchen and taking responsibility for what I put in my mouth. Then when I overate or ate wrong, how could it be my fault?

I was eating, ma'am, just eating what was available. And, of course, I was practicing good manners.

Who was I kidding? Only myself, it seemed.

It was no wonder then that our kitchen catered to my husband's taste and not mine. Last week, I ventured into the kitchen to make a batch of autumn chili and there wasn't any vinegar in the house. Andy was not a fan of chili, so why would he have a stash of vinegar? The *no chili blues* was the impetus for the flying journal words, *in my husband's kitchen.*

Shopping was a chore, not an event for me. My husband clipped his coupons and organized a weekly excursion. Andy has been known to be applauded at the checkout line for his coupon savings.

If I shopped again, I'd develop better eating habits. I'd make sugar-free gelatins, fat-burning bean soups and chilies, and maybe even a sheet of snickerdoodle cookies. They would make the house smell of Mom and cinnamon. No, it was not my mother's fault that I was fat, nor was it my husband's. It was mine and mine alone.

But I did need to stand up to them both and cook what I thrived upon and not what they thought was best. I knew my husband's feelings might get hurt, but he'd have to find someone else to feed. I thrived on protein and raw vegetables. Andy adored muffins, pasta, and cooked vegetables.

I'd make another appointment with the dietician. Armed with diabetic facts, I'd talk to Andy afterwards because the jig was up. I'd take responsibility for what I put in my mouth. Then I'd have no one to blame except myself if my blood sugar soared.

My mother's kitchen. My husband's kitchen. I needed Carole's kitchen. And, guess who had an unused kitchen in the upstairs unit of the double-decker? The excuse era was over. I biked home and made an appointment with a dietician.

The food pyramid had been shifting, plus I knew grains and bread weren't at the base of my personal pyramid as a result of Somersizing. While I was no longer Somersizing, I'd learned from Suzanne that vegetables and lots of them needed to be my base. Protein might be the second layer or perhaps low-fat milk and cottage cheese should be second. With the job change and moving, my weight had plateaued to a size eighteen. I was no longer losing weight. I had to work at maintaining the shedded pounds and proper blood sugar levels. I knew I needed to lose more, plus sugary foods still called to me. Perhaps they always would.

The dietician reviewed my food diary, which at least kept me honest and probably was the reason I hadn't gained weight. She was impressed with the completeness of my diary, but said I was making a mistake in one big area. She pulled out a carb chart.

"I want you to eat 45 grams of carb at breakfast and lunch and up to 75 grams at dinner," she said.

Me? Eat carbs?

"You can't be serious?" I questioned her. "You want me to eat three to five carb servings with every meal?"

"Yes," she smiled at me. "That amount will satisfy your brain and fill you up in a way that protein never will."

"You mean that I can eat a bagel again?" I flipped through the carb counts until I found the bagels. "I didn't think so. It says here that a bagel is 60 grams of carbs."

"A whole bagel is 60 grams." She took her plastic knife and cut a pretend bagel in two. "But, you can have a bagel, just not a whole one. A half is 30 grams."

"Really?"

"My grandmother always said," she paused for effect, "a lady only eats half of what's on her plate." She smiled. "My grandmother was ahead of her time."

"Grandmothers always are!" I meant it, too. My grandmother was ahead of her time knowing she needed a view and her art to remain interested in life. Plus, my grandmother had shown me what not to do when it came to eating. Now here was another grandmother teaching me another important lesson.

"Think in halves, not wholes. I like it," I said. "I'll try it."

My thin college roommate's voice echoed in my head. *Eat half of whatever is on your plate and dessert only once a week.* Patti certainly belonged to the Slim People's Club. Guess she had learned to be a lady early in life. Being a lady had never been my goal. But then, neither had being married. The female me said, *Carole might get it at last.*

"You can have half a bagel with an egg, a tablespoon of peanut butter, or a piece of cheese," the dietician brought me back to the discussion at hand. "A small apple can complete the breakfast."

"Sign me up."

I went home and changed how I kept my food diary. I began counting carbs, eating lots of veggies to fill up. I made up a list of food soothers. Celery with peanut butter. Turkey chili. Slices of lean meat wrapped around a pickle or lettuce leaves, lowfat yogurt laced with cottage cheese and sprinkled with almond slivers, tuna with cottage cheese and a half of a baked potato, or a whole sweet potato. Whoever thought a whole sweet potato was lower in carbs than an Idaho baked potato?

Then I had a heart-to-heart food talk with my husband. I was on a quest for an eating plan for life. Andy said he understood, but still stirred and baked his carb-loaded diet. Thankfully, he took his muffins and pasta salads to work. The staff loved him for it. And I loved that his goodies left the house.

I gave my second story refrigerator a complete makeover, inside and out. On the inside, I filled it with water bottles, cottage cheese, and vegetables. On the outside, I put favorite recipes. I joined Weight Watchers and learned about diet cola chicken, sugarless heavenly hash, and how to steam vegetables. Instead of being a source of temptation, my refrigerator became a good food buddy.

Embracing the kitchen at last, I made a place for myself in it. I could change as surely as the parkway changed with the seasons and be validated by low blood sugar readings. I could take charge of my eating as surely as I took charge of the Detroit hill biking all the way to the top. I could become Queen of the Mountain and the Kitchen. Maybe, I'll even forget about that outdated, pink Miss Piggy lunch box and buy an insulated lunch tote. Dr. Carey had been right in her first consultation with me. I needed to pack my lunch. And, when I arrived home, I needed to cook my dinner. Carole's Kitchen had blue, rather than creamy milk, oatmeal, apples, raw and frozen bags of naked vegetables, spices, sunflower seeds, and lots of protein. I liked the sound of it ... *In Carole's Kitchen*.

" Like the trees, we had to let each new year shape, teach, and renew us until our unconscious habits fell like autumn leaves to the forest floor, and new more conscious ways of doing things sprouted up in their place."
—Ken Carey from *Flat Rock Journal*

Chapter Twenty-One...Pink Slips

It was a white envelope, but it should have been pink. The envelope had been placed on the seat of my chair. Couldn't miss it. I picked it up, sat down, and opened it.

We regret to inform you that due to budgetary constraints, your employment has been terminated. Please see me at four to discuss the transition.

Me? Fired? What about my positive attitude and good work ethic? What about my promise to stay for the next ten years? What a way to tell a valued staff member that she is no longer needed. You're a chickenshit, Bob.

Nancy stuck her head in the door. "Are you ready for me?" Nancy was my first scheduled supervision of the day.

"Please come in." I tucked the letter in my daily planner and stuffed my personal feelings inside with it. I listened to Nancy's update on the children and families on her caseload. We discussed a few interventions that she might try with a mom who was beginning to trust her.

It was irrational to focus on the work at hand, but it quieted the screaming in my head.

How could he kick me out the door? Me? Of all people? I could think of a few people he should. And, of course, I thought about why hadn't I taken the other job where I would have been in charge four years ago instead of this one?

Sally came in next. She was no longer on my supervision list, but often ducked in to chat. She asked, "Will you be my supervisor again?"

"Why?"

"Linda's been let go." Sally threw her hands in the air. "How could Bob do that? If the chemo hasn't wiped her out, this will. How will she ever get health insurance?"

I'd heard commotion in the hall while I was seeing Nancy. Sally filled me in. "He not only let Linda go, but Anne's been let go, too."

"Well, you can add me to the list."

"What?" Sally's blue eyes grew huge.

"Yes. Me, too."

"Who'll supervise?"

"Guess Bob will."

"He can't do it all."

"Guess he thought this was the best way to get the budget in line. We all knew he had to do something." The rational part of my brain was functioning, even though I wanted to holler over and over, "Why me?"

Sally left to spread the news. By the morning's end, it was clear that Bob had laid off the entire, full-time supervisory tier of four, the two associate directors and two program directors. The uproar continued the rest of the day. Staff drifted in and out in two's and three's. They had solutions. They argued, "But we are a family here. We should have been asked for our ideas."

I thought back to my old regional director's job and the rage that I felt when I wasn't consulted and the big brothers and sisters were let go, indiscriminately. I continued to say to the staff that there was no meanness in this cut.

But, I resented doing Bob's work for him by sticking up for him. He'd created this mess and some lawyer must have instructed, make no unnecessary comments. He needed to meet with the four supervisors as a group and then with the staff to calm the case managers down. Instead, everyone was left to rant and stew while he was barricaded in his office behind closed doors.

I met with Bob at three.

"You must have known this was coming, Carole." Bob's eyes met mine. "It's no secret that the county child welfare budget is in serious trouble. They've cut every agency's fees."

"I knew that you needed to do something, but I feel blindsided."

"I can't keep everybody. I prayed on it." He shuffled some papers on his desk. "I've done all the supervision before."

"Yes. And that's why you hired me."

"I appreciate what you have done." He smiled at me. "With your reputation you'll have no trouble finding a position."

I didn't answer that volley. I wasn't up to making him feel better. I did discuss with him my job priorities for the rest of the week.

During the last week, I worked hard finishing reports and upcoming staff evaluations. I left on Friday afternoon with everyone's best wishes, my unused vacation days, and a severance package of four weeks. One week for every year that I'd worked for the agency.

The next morning, I dragged myself out of bed. Ran a brush through my hair. Put on a touch of lipstick. No need yet to look like the unwashed, frumpy Michael Keaton in *"Mr. Mom."* Last night's dinner conversation was still playing in my head.

"I haven't been without a job since age 14," I said. "And, I've never been fired."

"You were not fired," lectured my husband over dinner. "You were laid off."

"Laid off is too polite a word for what happened," I retorted. "I was fired."

Andy knew better than to say more. But, in a way, he was right. I'd need to get past my anger. I needed some perspective. I needed to stay pulled together. Thank God for my morning practices of biking and journaling. My morning routine had not been disturbed. Nor would they be because I had a life now, beyond work.

I poked my head in my second story studio. Outside, a jagged yellow streak of sun had risen out of a clam shell sky. No rain yet. Swirling autumn winds were at play, beckoning me. I greeted Andy in the kitchen, where he was sipping coffee and reading the newspaper. I donned my whistle and bike helmet.

I rolled my bike out of the garage and rode down the street to the top of the hill leading into the Valley Parkway. The clam shell sky snapped shut. The jagged band of sunlight was locked away, inaccessible. The northern winds hit me in the face, arms, and chest as I began my descent. I could hardly stay upright. I dismounted and walked my bike down the hill as seeds, leaves, and twigs assaulted me. The wind roared at me. *Enough already!*

I roared back letting my stuffed feelings explode. "I know you. So you want to play rough?"

At the bottom of the hill, I mounted my bike giving my handbrakes a couple of squeezes. I was ready. The pathway was littered with fall debris. A glob of debris clapped me on the back, taunting me.

"Let the wild rumpus begin." I was one with the elements and the Parkway. I rode and rode. The wind ran with me shrieking through the trees making gusts of fall confetti to rain upon me. Finally out of breath, I stopped and pushed my bike down a path to the Rocky River. Above me, I watched but could barely hear the jet planes from Hopkins straining to climb through the fossilized clouds. Today was a day to stay on the ground. The birds knew that. They chirped at me from safe corners of nature. None of them were flying around today unlike me and my emotions.

The Rocky River churned into brown froth. I was a child again throwing rocks and sticks into the river chanting, "Sink or swim." I was a child again jumping in leaf piles breathing in bits of leaves and stored sunlight. I was a child again hearing the chain hitting the flagpole of the schoolyard of my childhood. I didn't see a flagpole, but saw, instead, blue hooded boats on dry land hunkered down for the winter in the curve of a hill. Their lines sang in the wind as they slapped their sides.

I didn't need coffee today as nature had already jolted me wide-awake. I trudged up the hill pushing my bike out of the valley feeling spent, yet satisfied having danced to the drumbeats of the war dance below.

As I opened my journal at the Borderline Café, I felt restored, and at peace. I'd record nature's fall fury that had suited me so well. I'd store it deep inside beside the flagpole rallying sound of my youth reminding me that life's dance is waiting within, waiting for me to "Come out and play." And in the end, a warm meal would be spread before me.

Before I left on my wild bike ride, I'd tucked Carole's Diabetic Prediction Path (CDPP) into my journal to review over breakfast. I was ready now to create Carole's Fired Prediction Path (CFPP).

It took a week of steady thinking but at the end of it, I had a workable plan.

Carole's Fired Prediction Path (CFPP)

Behavior / Feeling Challenge: Scared

Trigger	Intervention	Do Now	Life-Long
Monthly bills come in.	Stick to budget. Find a temp job.	Exercise the demons away.	As long as willing to work, income is possible.

"No Job" anxiety.	Send out 2 resumes, and make one cold call per week.	Make a list of where want to work.	Satisfying work is always available.
Rejection Letters. No Leads.	Take an interesting course. Learn a new skill.	Journal. Send thank you note for being considered.	Pray. Ask for blessings.

Behavior / Feeling Challenge: Feeling Deprived

Trigger	Intervention	Do Now	Life-Long
Pity Party Day.	Don't soothe with sugary foods.	Use CDPP.	Record blessings in a journal.
When job doesn't appear overnight.	Treat self kindly.	Go to ER Shelves: gum, bubble bath, film.	Read good book. Visit a library, zoo, museum.
When want to go shopping.	Organize closets. *New look* finds.	Access *rainy day* fun fund.	Find a project. Volunteer.

Behavior / Feeling: Frustrated

Trigger	Intervention	Do Now	Life-Long
Severance runs out.	Stick to job plan.	Sign up for unemployment.	Believe in self. Know another door will open.
Nothing in sight.	Stick to job plan. Network. Stay in professional loop. Be visible.	Go for a bike ride. Set up lunch date with a colleague.	Remember: Nature heals. *Valley Parkway, Here I come.*

Having a plan made me feel better, but I remained worried. I was nearing sixty and couldn't promise anyone ten years anymore, or could I? What was so magical about age, 65? But I had to face it. I was in a tough age bracket to be hired into middle management. I had my art and it did supplement, but couldn't support paying the mortgage on the double decker house and the final years of the kids' college loans. I needed work unless I moved my office to the basement and we rented the top half of the house out. Whenever I thought about that possibility, my heart stopped.

Thank God, I had at least a severance package and could enroll in Andy's health plan as a spouse. Fleeting thoughts of using my savings and severance pay for travel entered my mind. Look how Vegas had refreshed me. *See something new. But...but...Carole, now is not a good time to spend money. I whined.*

There were other ways to see something new. *Just look at anything differently, Carole.* The Valley Parkway and all its seasons was there for me to explore at my new leisure. And, I did. It always lifted my spirits and got my endorphins charged up.

Good writing also improved my vision. One day digging in my *keeper* essay file, I rediscovered the Abbott article that I'd read in Vegas. In an interview in *Publishers Weekly*, author Shirley Abbott wrote: "Every age has to redefine its reality, that's what writers and historians are about; we're all revisionists...To look at your life in this way is a way of creating it, a way of controlling it, so that the mythology shall spring from the life and not the life from the mythology."

Shirley Abbott was a memoir writer. In her first book, she'd delved into the relationship of mothers and daughters. In another book, she shared the heritage that her father had handed her. I devoured memoirs for I was as drawn to reading them as I'd once been to eating popcorn. The salty taste of memoirs lingers in kernels of truth that pop open one's life such as: "Every age has to redefine reality."

Now Abbott's use of age had more to do with the historic period of a person's lifetime, but for me the micro meaning of age as being one's current numerical birthday arrested me now just as it had in Vegas. In Vegas, I'd started sorting out my life realizing that I was enmeshed in a full blown, mid-life crisis triggered by the diagnosis of diabetes, the death of my mother, and the children leaving town. I'd met midlife head-on by making many changes. I ate differently. I didn't collapse into a recliner every night. I took a manageable administrative job so that I could have a life after work. I felt and acknowledged my feelings, honoring them. I renewed my artist vows. I was writing again.

Now that I was almost sixty and *fired*, what myths did my life hold and how were these myths shaping me now rather than me shaping the myths myself? As a second story woman, I needed a second story to tell myself. But first I had to clear-cut more old myths as a logger does in the North Woods. Why is it that old beliefs die hard and keep sprouting up again?

Did I really believe that if I didn't work a sixty-hour work week, that I was not a good employee?

Did I really believe that I'd brought this firing on myself just as I'd believed that I had caused my diabetes? Shame on me!

Did I really believe that I could write full-time and support myself?

Did I really believe that having a view was everything? Was I willing to give it up?

Did I believe that role models for life after sixty were only Sun City, snowbirds, and reading my eyes out? Could retirement be a big hoax? Could life after sixty be a whole new creative era?

I felt better asking these questions and pondering answers. I needed to understand the myths that defined the first half of my life so that I could imagine the myths that would dominate the second half. In the first half of life, I'd been an over-achiever. But my archenemy, diabetes, had forced me to a halt. I'd taken a long look at my life while in Las Vegas and didn't like what I saw. I always wanted to be a leader, *important*, and do good works. In doing so, I'd drawn hellish *to do* lists and fled from dreaded introspection. I was in permanent flight from myself, wanting to get it all done—all done to the point that I didn't know what all done was. I'd focused on anything and everything but me and kept on doing so. It had become a habit for me to find a cause, a worthy direction to pursue.

I made a new *to do* list of what I wanted to do now that I was fired. As an effective parent educator, I'd develop a list of trainings and send it out to area agencies and the surrounding child welfare departments. I'd do this despite the fact that training calendars were set up a year in advance in October and I'd been let go in November. The timing was bad, but they might need a fill-in or a substitute.

I'd also been a solid field supervisor for social work students. I'd write the college and see if they needed a field liaison for a cohort of field supervisors for the coming year. I'd start my Second Chance Vegas book that I was always talking about writing. There was an editorial nibble on a children's book that I was rewriting.

I settled into a routine. Lined up some trainings. The professor of field placements responded: *Nothing is available at this time. We'll keep your resume on file.* A week later she phoned, asking, "Carole, would you be on the field instruction advisory committee?"

I said, "Yes." *Get your name out there, Carole. Volunteer. Mingle.*

I settled into *Carole's Fired Prediction Path.* And on days when all seemed hopeless, I roared down the Valley Parkway trails singing my own tune. "She'll be coming around the mountain when she comes. She'll be coming around the mountain she comes."

"Hope is the thing with feathers
That perches in the soul,
And sings the tune without the words,
And never stops at all."
    —Emily Dickinson

Chapter Twenty-Two...How Wonderful!

I couldn't help but think that "being laid off" was not unlike last April's snowstorm. Spring had officially arrived heralded by the return of the robins and bursting forsythia. Then, without warning, a winter storm came thundering across Lake Erie out of the northeast. I, on my bike, and the migratory robins were mesmerized by its fury. Me, by choice, and they with no choice but to endure.

Pushing my bike along a two-foot, plushy carpeted snow trail, I saw a robin clinging to an icy branch in my camera frame. He didn't move, hunkered deep into an inner hearth. Cold or maybe feet frozen stiff, he didn't move anything but his eyes at my approach to capture him on film. He was ready for spring rains and worms, but instead, the rewards for flying hard to reach his summer home were snow, slim pickings, and a silly photographer.

After taking his portrait, I bowed to thank him. His eyes remained glued on me as I withdrew and put my camera carefully away from the elements. He had given me a wondrous gift. Photography is like that. One never knows where one will find a soulful image. Posting his photo on the refrigerator last April as a possible Christmas card, this robin has emerged instead as a daily reminder to "keep the faith." Spring would come just as another job would. After all, licensed social workers, like registered nurses, never have to worry about finding work because there are always more jobs than trained professionals available. However, I wasn't sure (or broke enough yet) that I wanted to go back to having a caseload and a 24/7 beeper.

The holidays were coming and I was two weeks into being terminated, but "Not dead yet, thank you very much!" (I had been re-reading Carolyn See, author of *Making A Literary Life,* and had adopted her "rejection is a process" sarcasm.) Wanting to create some extra cash, I signed up for a craft show that had an opening.

After setting up, I donated a box of photo cards at the organizer's table. Door prizes were solicited from the participating artists hoping to draw the crowd to their table. Unfortunately, there wasn't much of a crowd that Saturday, but I had some good early sales despite the sparse customer base.

Many of the artists were grumbling, crossing this show off their list for next year. I needed to stay "up" and not get caught in this negative thinking. Giving myself a pep talk, I remembered an artist friend's advice about being generous at shows. She had said, "Then goodness will flow back to you in unexpected ways."

I purchased a few gifts from neighboring tables and bartered trades with interested artists. Feeling the ions changing around me, I gave twenty dollars away purchasing 24 door prize tickets. It was for a good cause as the funds were going to a domestic violence shelter.

The announcement for the first drawing came over the loud speaker. "Would Carole Calladine please pick up a door prize?"

The prize was a beautiful, hand-thrown bowl painted in turquoise and tan. I'd purchased a mug earlier from the same artist. I was thrilled.

A half-hour later, the organizer announced another raffle ticket winner. "Would Carole Calladine please pick up a door prize?"

I'd won a hand-dipped, chunky candle on a snowflake plate, a perfect holiday centerpiece.

By the time the next door prize was announced, my fellow vendors were kidding me about the drawing being fixed. And so they should have. Probably because the traffic was sparse and raffle sales minimal, I won seven prizes including a hand-dyed scarf, a kaleidoscope, and crystal earrings. I left the craft show feeling flush. Besides the prizes, I'd had respectable sales and purchased and bartered for several pleasing works of art. After participating in a one-day holiday craft boutique, I was set for the upcoming gift giving season.

What an amazing way to start the holiday! I felt relieved of holiday shopping and hassling the crowds. Plus, I wasn't carrying a 24/7 crisis beeper, the bane of a social worker's existence. How relaxing! How refreshing in contrast to other holiday years when I'd often run frantically around staying on top of social work brush fires, buying last minute gifts, and creating personal debt.

After the holiday season passed, I received a few "parent education" bookings. Then a fellow artist and shop owner asked me to convene a 12-week course using Julia Cameron's *The Artist's Way.*

Why not? I had the time and lesson plans since I'd taught this class before. It would be fun to introduce others to the magic of reconnecting to the creative source. Plus, maybe this review would do me some good on my current journey. I desperately wanted to believe, "Leap and the net will appear." Even though it felt like, "Pushed and will my parachute open?"

About six weeks into teaching from *The Artist's Way*, Mary Sue from my old agency came calling to take me to lunch. She had been instructed to lure me back as a consultant to the regional director. At the same time, a competing agency's director also phoned having heard that I wasn't on vacation, but had been laid off.

The word was out. Did you hear that Carole Calladine was laid off? I was never comfortable when questioned about the dismissal. One part of me was embarrassed and another part of me was angry. How could anyone lay me off? So when asked, I got good at saying in a matter-of-fact tone and sticking to the facts, "Yes, I was laid off due to budgetary constraints." I immediately followed that statement by, "Know of any good jobs?" That put everyone at ease, including me.

The second agency offering me a job was in audit trouble. Both agencies were offering administrative positions with no cut in salary. So much for collecting unemployment benefits and being too old to find a management job in social work. And here, I'd begun to believe that I was being given a chance in life to collect unemployment and be a starving artist. A part of me had been secretly pleased about joining the ranks of Broadway dancers and actors between shows.

Now, it was decision time because I couldn't collect unemployment if I was being offered a job. And if I couldn't collect unemployment, would I have to rent the top half of our double out? That might force the question of which offer should I take? Then again, maybe I shouldn't take either one. Should I keep developing my writing and photography skills and count on enlarging my parent education training base to pay the mortgage? A free-lance lifestyle was appealing. But a job offered income security and continued studio occupancy of the upstairs unit. What did I want to be when I grew up all over again?

I kept remembering a good friend's response to my being laid off.

"How wonderful!" she'd said. I was glad we were on the phone so I didn't have to disguise my face into a mask to cover the hurt I was feeling. How could my friend think this was wonderful, unless she wasn't truly a friend?

"Wonderful?" I asked.

"Well, Carole. You know you never would have quit." She paused, "Wait till you see what's in store for you now."

My upset quieted. This friend really believed in me! Probably more than I did. Would I wait and see what was in store for me? Or, did I want more of the same, familiar work?

The line staff at my old agency placed a few calls to me. "Please come back. We miss you."

I told both agencies that I needed a week to think about their offer. While thinking, I read portions of favorite memoirs for insight. A friend suggested a new book, *The Heroine's Journey* by Maureen Murdock. In this book, Murdock, a psychotherapist, talked about how successful women were often "daughters of the father." They had felt accepted by their dads and therefore, accepted by the culture in a patriarchal system. That was me. Dad, Big Daddy, and Jens Juhl (my Bestafa) had been my champions.

Murdock's words echoed true inside of me. I'd played by the men's rules and had risen to the top of my profession. I'd changed from being a nurturing therapist and gone into administration. I was into system issues, "big" issues having put aside the feminine energy it takes to be a full-time "caring" therapist.

The switch gave me a chance to use my skills to supervise and teach. And, it gave me a leadership role to challenge system issues, which eventually had consumed me. That's a huge part of why I'd taken a mid-management role. I wanted a *life* outside of social work. My body demanded it. Some say diabetes was a symptom of needing more sweetness in one's life. That sweetness for me was found in photography, writing, and taking the time to live mindfully. I rode my bike daily to feel the wind on my face and feel the pen move across the pages of my journal.

Murdock said, women on *The Heroine's Journey* must heal the body and soul as well as the mind. Women must accept the feminine as well as the masculine parts of themselves. I guess—no, I know now—that I really needed to see those Vegas showgirls. I needed to be at peace with my soft, curvy body. I needed to come full circle in my belly dance so I could understand the quote engraved on a rock outside the gates of Lakeside, the community that had become one of my favorite retreat places. "We shall not cease from exploration and the end of all our exploring will be to arrive where we started and know the place for the first time, through the unknown, remembered gate when the last of earth left to discover is that which was the beginning..." T. S. Eliot

Had I come full circle and knew it for the first time? Was I able to act on one of Murdock's guiding principles? "Women today are acquiring the courage to express their vision, the strength to set limits, and the willingness to take responsibility for themselves and others in a new way." I was open to a new way.

In *The Artist's Way* class, we were on an image quest. In one exercise, Cameron suggested that recovering artists start an image file. "List five desires...be alert for images of these desires. When you spot them, clip them, buy them, photograph them, draw them, *collect them somehow*. With these images, begin a file of dreams that speak to you." Participants were making important self-discoveries.

I joined in. Tearing images and words from magazines, finding postcards, and sorting through a photo stash, I put these treasures in a box. Then I intoned a prayer of intention in my journal asking for guidance about my career choices.

The next morning, I lifted the lid on the box, plucking a baker's dozen from within. I wrote down first thoughts, uncensored thoughts.

1. The affirmation, "I am enough."
Yes, I am. And whatever I decide, I don't have to work a 70-hour-work week for approval and to stay employed.

2. A cowboy with an attitude lounging against a fence.
What would this bad girl choose now that I'd been told to, "Get out of Dodge."?

3. A picture depicting the sacrifice of Isaac.
Wait! A sacrifice of your beloved, isn't required. I can heal myself whole without amputating a limb, or a family member, or sweetness from my life. Go now, with God's blessing.

4. A photo of a dragon imprinted on a bowl.
Share your fire, Dragon. How should I fill this empty bowl that the firing kiln has made strong and ready for use?

5. Norman Rockwell painting a self-portrait.
I identified with Norman looking in a mirror and painting himself on canvas. "Stick your neck out, too, Carole. Write a memoir."

6. A photo of Tambora's volcano, a crater that is three miles wide.
Words from the accompanying article in National *Geographic Magazine* had caught my eye. Mary Shelley, who wrote the entertaining classic, *Frankenstein*, wanted it to serve "as a warning not to overlook the consequences of humanity's tampering with nature."

I renewed my soul's desires when my personal volcano of diabetes erupted and released the demons within. I was rewriting the truths and lies in my life, restoring my natural optimism and good nature.

7. "You rise by lifting others." Robert Green Ingersoll.

Teaching lifts others. So does art. So does social work. I will rise sending meaningful smoke signals from inner, smoldering embers.

8. An image of a matchbook cover advertising David Mamet's *The Old_Neighborhood*. The under flap read, "Close cover before striking."

Strike out in a new direction, Carole. Mamet won the Pulitzer. Blow your cover as a closet writer.

9. "Youth is a quality, not a matter of circumstances." Frank Lloyd Wright.

Old age is a quality, too, and not a matter of circumstances. What circumstances did I want to pursue, regardless of age? What had my experience taught me?

10. A child hiding behind a towel looking contrite, saying, "I didn't do it."

I didn't do what? I didn't want to be 90 (my Dad's age) and have any regrets about what I did or didn't do.

11. A poster, "Show postponed."

You don't have to take these first job offers. You can leap and the net will appear in time.

12. At age 89, Helen Levitt's fifth book of photographs are published depicting NY curbsides, stoops, fire escapes, and people going about their daily lives.

Artists never lose interest in living well. I must remain an artist.

13. A woman dressed in pure white. Headline screams: "Nix Your Fix." "Liberate yourself from the power of passive addiction: beer, chocolate, and cigarettes. Natural remedies can help you take back control."

White ashes rain down on me, the original work-a-holic who burned herself, inside out. I can reinvent myself.

The 13 images spoke. I couldn't believe how many images spoke of *fire* to me. *How wonderful!* I thought. *What marvelous things were in store for me if I was brave enough to strike out in new directions? Could I get beyond my automatic protection mode? Did I have the courage to not try, try, try again but try something different?*

I'd been put in the controlled burn area feeling scorched ever since Bob cut the middle management staff to hose down the out of control budget. Mid-management was always the first cut. I had vowed to never accept another mid-management position. That left bohemian artist, director, or direct service line staff. I knew I'd be good as a service provider as I had considerable social work skills. But what about other smoldering passions of writing, teaching, and photography? What would happen to them? They were the new growth areas in me. Where was the fearless Vegas traveler?

It was time to unleash the dragon, ignite its fire, blazing a new trail. I was ready to climb aboard. Thus, I made my first decision with ease.

I told Mary Sue, "No." I knew in my heart that I couldn't go backwards. But I did give the current regional director a list of suggestions to strengthen their recruiting base. He thanked me and probably breathed a sigh of relief because his job was secure for the moment. Plus, if I'd learned anything in this life, it was not to burn any bridges in case the new path was a dead end.

Breathing easier myself, I turned to the agency in audit trouble. My colleagues warned: "Don't work for them. You have your reputation to look after." But they hadn't seen my image box and I didn't tell them about, "Get out of Dodge." I'd always wanted to be a bad girl, but had been too uptight to be one.

My colleagues would think I'd lost it. And if they knew about my image box, they'd probably interpret the signs differently using Jungian theory to support their opinions and confuse me.

Instead, I listened to my gut. The images were not only loaded with *fire* signs, they spoke of a new kind of firing to me. My wise husband had been wrong and I was right. I hadn't been laid off, I'd been fired; fired up to do new things.

My second decision was that I refused the audit-troubled agency's management offer. Instead, I proposed that I become a part-time, training director to meet head-on their deficiencies, designing a trainer-of-the-trainer series for their seven offices, statewide. Then, I went on about my business. If they bought it, they bought it. If they didn't, another open door would appear. I couldn't quite believe my audacity but it had certainly felt good to feel in charge of my work choices.

I continued to line up training gigs, facilitate *The Artist's Way*, ride my bike, and write. Now was the time to live fully the lessons gleaned from my disease. The thirteen fire images kept reinforcing the change that I was seeking in earning a living. I'd allow my artistic passions to erupt, spill over, and follow the lava flowing in new directions.

I didn't have to wait long for an offer from the second agency. Within the month, I accepted a part-time position as a training director at a generous hourly rate. (If I worked a 20-hour week, I would make what I used to make as a full-time, salaried professional.) Plus, this work assignment was a win/win situation. The agency needed shoring up and I wanted to garner more training experience. I settled in. The staff more than accepted me, particularly after I set up a successful meeting that lifted the hold on the agency. The local child welfare agency would again place children with them accepting the corrective action plan. My reputation had preceded me.

By early summer, the field placement professor phoned from the social work department of a local college. A resignation by a part-time, field liaison had been turned in. "Are you still available for the next school year, Carole?"

"Yes." *I couldn't believe my good fortune.*

At the end of the summer, an introductory, social work course at the university needed an instructor. "Carole, are you available?"

"Yes." I pinched myself. I wasn't dreaming.

I was becoming the dream itself. The image quest was becoming true. I was striking out in new directions having found a new vision of myself. I knew this wasn't the final chapter in earning a living, but I also knew that finding a full-time job would scare me. I might lose myself again. Or, live in fear that the last hired was the first one out when the budget needed to be cut. Wanting to surround myself with options, I had done so. I'd nixed my fix and become the dragon in charge of my work day.

"Thank you, Bob, for firing me. How else could this have ever happened? How wonderful!"

A new world opened up. Wings against a blue sky fluttered inside of me singing words of thanksgiving. The freezing robin clinging to the branch had thawed and been freed by the fires lit from within.

" There is a garden in every childhood, an enchanted place where colors are brighter, the air softer, and the morning more fragrant than ever before."
—Elizabeth Lawrence

Chapter Twenty-Three...Emerald Necklace Hosannas

The March morning was cold, but the four-note trills of the chickadees welcomed the cat and me as we poked our heads out the side door at six a.m. Time for me to ride in the parkway while the cat went to patrol his back yard. I coasted down Rockcliff Road on my bike listening to the sounds of the woods' overture warming up for the day ahead. For ten years now, I have been riding my bike and I still never knew what gifts the Emerald Necklace Parkland would reveal on any given day. Change was always present with no two days alike.

Today the ground on the walking trails along the Rocky River was polished to a buff tan. Individual leaves were emerging from their icy mud baths, drained of their fall color. A fallen tree, pushed and pulled by rushing water was temporarily beached on an ancient, lippy road spanning the Rocky River. Hung up by its roots, the three-inch, raised cement sides of the road held fast onto the tree. Only tomorrow, or the next day, would tell the story of whether the river rose and dislodged the tree, or whether the tree's roots tore the lip holding it, or if another fallen tree rammed into it, jarring it loose. Or perhaps, a fisherman, whose lines became entangled in the roots, would hack at the tree, freeing its body to slip over the old road on its journey to Lake Erie.

As I biked on, I stopped to photograph the wrinkled skins of the winterized trees. They reminded me of unboiled prunes hardened into gnarled grooves. Soon, however, their inner sap would gush forth and flow to the very tips of their branches. They'd leaf and this greening would fill the woods with delicious spring and I'd sing my hosannas of renewal with them.

Good reading has this same effect on me filling me with hosannas. Recently I'd rediscovered A. A. Milne's tales of *Winnie-The-Pooh.*

Pooh, like I, had gotten himself in a tight place. Pooh always liked a little something at eleven o'clock in the morning, and when Rabbit said, "Honey or condensed milk with your bread?" he was so excited that he said, "Both." Well you can imagine what happened next. He ate so much he couldn't pass through Rabbit's doorway, even with Rabbit pushing Pooh from behind with his strong legs. He was stuck fast, unable to enter or leave. Rabbit had to fetch Christopher Robin who said: "Silly old Bear. We shall have to wait for you to get thin again. I'm afraid no meals. But we will read to you."

So for a week Christopher Robin read Pooh a Sustaining Book, such as would help and comfort a Wedged Bear in Great Tightness,...

Afterwards, Winnie-The-Pooh was pulled *free* by his friends just as morning practices and my artist friends have sustained and pulled the new me free. *Have I learned my lesson or do I still need oodles of honey and milk with my bread?* I liked to think that I was no longer a silly old bear. After all, at the beginning of this journey, the bear in Vegas had urged me to find the "just right experience." And, I'd been working on this task ever since.

My journals bulged with the "just right experiences." I'd learned tasty, new eating habits. I liked a fresh catawba melon or raspberries for sweets. I liked a steamed medley of zucchini, broccoli, and onion over brown rice with a sprinkling of parmesan cheese. I liked a moist turkey meatloaf basted with chicken broth. I liked a bowl of oatmeal with blueberries, cinnamon and skim milk. I liked the texture of a crisp salad of naked, mixed greens. I liked being awake and alive again without overeating on sugary desserts in the first half of my life. All those "just desserts" piled on the weight and pushed the snooze button in my head.

I'd have a bowl of ice cream and cake or pie, eating at my leisure in front of the television in a darkened family room until I was sporting my grandmother's contented Buddha belly leaving my mother's athletic body behind and losing any chance of an enlightened, Buddha mind. The cares and interactions of the day fell off of me with every mouthful. I feasted myself into a sleepy bliss only to get up the next day, fatigued, and live that day just as hard and just as unprocessed as the one before. This was living? I think not. This was one version of what the experts called burn-out. And its side effect for me was eating myself into a disability.

I'd learned to get off my duff and find exercises that I liked. Biking in the out-of-doors remained at the top of my list. Anything out-of-doors revived my body and spirits. I even had a gym membership now to tone and strengthen my upper body, although I still wasn't wearing lycra.

I still had weight to lose, but had kept off what I'd lost. I could shop in regular clothing stores now. My doctor continued to work with me, even though I wasn't a model patient. I have had backslides, but she gave me credit for the changes that I'd made and waited for me to get back on track. That belief has helped me. Neither of us had thrown in the towel and said, "What's the use?" I was still managing my diabetes with diet, exercise, and medication. We both knew that everything counted in staying healthy with this disease.

I had diabetes along with 230 million people worldwide or more specifically the 21 million people in the United States. Ninety percent of us had Type 2. However I looked at it, I was one of millions who ate too much and exercised too little, complicating my body's struggle with too much fat.

Diabetes was a set-up and one of its pronounced symptoms was feeling hungry all the time, especially after eating. In simple terms, the body was made up of millions of cells nourished by food broken down into a sugar, or glucose. This sugar was transported by the blood and blood vessels to the cells to use as energy. Only in diabetes, the glucose couldn't get in. The result was that the sugar levels rise, yet the cells were still hungry sending signals to the brain for more food. *More food, please.*

Diabetes was certainly a creepy disease. Clogging blood streams with thick, sugary sludge, slowly damaged the body. Heart attacks, foot amputations, getting hung up on the lip of a submerged road were the unseen bottom line. Rushing around eating whatever was handy for a little pick-me-up created a perfect body environment for diabetes to flourish.

I couldn't erase having this chronic disease. It was present in my body. But I knew that I'd discovered how to be kind to my diabetic body through morning practices and self-monitoring. I could strengthen my body by scheduled, structured acts of kindness. Whether or not my body continued to respond with lowered blood sugar readings and weight loss was not the issue here. The issue was that I'd shown up. I moved my bike across the metro park pathways and my pen across the tabletops of the Borderline café. I'd stood up and made myself accountable.

This showing up had gone a long way in nurturing my mature body and psyche. It'd separated the disease into two syllables. I was no longer at dis-ease with my mind and body. Instead, I was at-ease. Every time, every day that I honored my body and mind through the ritual of morning practices, I was being considerate and building confidence within myself. The answer to diabetes, life's losses, and burn-out was so simple and so complex at the same time.

1. Stop, listen, and look. Take a time-out for good behavior and do nothing. Relax.
2. Journal. Process the day, fleeting thoughts, and feelings. Become Buddha calm and enlightened.
3. Exercise. Bodies feel loved when muscles are flexed and used.
4. Eat for nourishment rather than dying to get to the next ice cream stand.
5. Find life-sustaining friends who inspire living creatively and with passion.
6. Repeat affirmations such as *I am enough* throughout the day and pray for spiritual deliverance when getting in *too tight* places.
7. Keep emergency shelves stocked with good ideas and "rainy day" soothers.
8. Use the Prediction Path when ambushed by behaviors and feelings that triggered a setback. Build confidence by addressing the setback and recover by keeping the faith through healthy interventions.
9. Remember that diabetes, or any other chronic condition, never goes on a holiday; but I can and I will.

Diabetes had been my wake-up call. I not only changed my diet and recliner activities, I sought out new sweetness in life and found it in photography, social work that compliments my skills and lifestyle, and in Artist Way friendships.

Why just yesterday, I'd come home from work and found two baskets of violas resting at my back door. I touched the velvet orange petals, one of the first flowers able to be planted and survive a cold, northern spring. I brought them inside to the sunroom porch. I wouldn't take any chances. I'd wait a couple more weeks before I planted them at my side door to greet me first thing in my comings and goings.

Phoning Shirley, a member of my Artist Way (AW) cluster group, I asked, "You wouldn't know anything about a good fairy leaving violas on my doorstep?"

"I've never been a good fairy before."

"You just made my day."

"They looked like you."

They looked like me. Now was that a friend or what?

Our AW cluster continued to meet monthly. Every woman in it hugged herself embracing the friendships forged there as we journeyed into who we wanted to be in the second half of life. Every meeting we had "show and tell." We "showed off" and were applauded by our AW sisterhood. First efforts, as well as fully blossomed projects were respected. Honored. We were alive and growing our talents.

Shirley, mother of two, grandmother of four, was not only a good fairy, but was Joseph of the many-colored coat. I envied her enthusiasm for living well and tried to emulate, rather than be outright jealous.

I needed to keep learning from this friend because *Shirley* was— what I wasn't, wanted to be, and may never be—a bohemian artist who knew how to effortlessly create homemade abundance in life. I continually marveled at her generosity, spontaneity, and flexibility in welcoming treasures into her life.

Artist boutiques had begged Shirley for years to let them sell her original designer jackets and bags. But Shirley wasn't interested in creating to sell. Instead, down-sized from her company's training department, she took her 401 K and only used some of the interest as income. She became a free spirit, finding extra work to learn something new or to help a friend. Money never seemed to be a consideration.

I kidded her often. "You are a migrant worker, Shirley. The only difference is that you have a fully-paid home waiting for you at all times."

Often, I was filled with "a longing" admiration.

Shirley facilitated sewing classes, teaching and learning with the participants. Open to adventures, Shirley struck up a conversation with a national fabric artist at the sewing store who needed a helper at a state exhibition. The artist ended up not only paying Shirley's way, but gave my friend a huge product discount from a sponsoring fabric company.

If I was Shirley, I just knew that I could become a bohemian writer —wearing funky clothes and living on the edge of nowhere. But, I wasn't that brave yet.

You might find Shirley as the cashier at an auction, in the greenhouse of a friend on a weekend, or babysitting the backstage door of a national touring company. Watch out for the Shirley's of the world. Their freeing magic would change the face of retirement if others caught on to new ways of living. And, if you are fortunate to have a friend like Shirley, you never knew what you'd find on your doorstep.

I've learned a lot from Shirley and all AW friends, but I've especially learned to be a better me, to have fun in the present moment, and that earning a living was all around you for the taking. They were reminders that one can get too busy earning a living instead of building a rich, "happily ever after" life in your fifties, sixties, and seventies. What would Shirley and my friends teach me in our eighties?

My AW friends were there to emulate, cheer, and model living well creatively. They cushioned the aftermath of life's inevitable losses. Sustaining losses of family, health, work were easier if fortunate enough to be surrounded by such a circle of sistership. These friends gave me a sense of place. A Harvard researcher has said, "Contrary to popular belief, girls are not just standing on the sidelines of the playground. They are practicing lifelong conversations with friends." Wanting sustenance in my life, I found girlfriends again.

I'd forgotten how narrow my life had become without playmates. My friend, Mary had died. Other good friends had also been lost through moves, divergent interests, divorce, and more deaths. At fifty, I'd ballooned up with "all work and no play." Work had become my other family, which was never a good idea.

An artist friend, Muriel, who had moved to Oklahoma, continued to stay in touch. After reading an essay or two from shared journal writings, she wrote me. "I can really remember how you enjoyed rich tasty foods. You also like rich color, texture as well as people and places that appealed to the senses. Some people just are more sensual."

I quarreled with Muriel in my head. How dare she see me as more sensual than average. *What? Me, sensual? After all, I was a social worker and not a Vegas showgirl. That was a laughable idea, wasn't it?* I'd tossed that letter into my notebook and forgot about it. I came across it recently reviewing journals from this decade's journey.

Now I see that Muriel saw me more clearly than I'd seen myself. I'd never thought of myself as being sensual at my very core. After all, I was midwestern sturdy, grounded in reality, working hard as a social worker, and didn't bruise easily. Or, was I being bruised repeatedly adding layer after layer of insulating fat protecting myself from the pain of others and disconnecting myself from my true nature? I knew the answer now to that question and to the question of—*How can you be so cold?*

Thinking back on my resilient social work career, the "a-ha" light exploded in my mind. I'd constantly taken on lots and overwhelmed myself. Constantly addressing and fixing work challenges, I'd become restless and bored, and then move on to another job—until my last assignment as an assistant director. There I'd protected and crafted a life outside of work. I needed to thank Bob for those four years. I always thrived on doing good with my life, not worried about doing well. Social workers prided themselves on getting a higher education to advocate for others. I'd needed a new message. *Be good to myself, refresh myself, and I will work well.*

Riding the all-purpose trails in the Emerald Necklace woods on a freshly cleansed Easter morning, the light was heaven sent. I felt blessed by its radiance especially after enduring five straight days of gray rain. Ralph Waldo Emerson must have experienced such light when he wrote the line, "The sky is the daily bread of the eyes."

The ground was covered with wild flowers whose names I knew and more laid hidden in patches of beauty in the woods. Purple flowering myrtle, stalks of bluebells, and dainty dogtooth violets lifted their heads in a sun dance. The pileated woodpecker, red head bobbing, beat out a drum tattoo with his black beak on the side of a tall pin oak while the northern cardinal broke into a three-note trill. I stopped and we whistled back and forth to one another while the woodpecker's tattoo beat accompanied us. I couldn't help but grin. *Ewa-yea! Minne-wawa!*

I stopped at the bridge and stared into the water, daydreaming, enjoying a moment of grace. A throaty clicking noise caught my attention pulling me back to the present. Some pebbles plopped into the river. I stayed still spotting the telltale ripples in the water. A raccoon peeked her vigilant nose out a drainpipe and detecting no motion led her young ones into the shade of the bridge to cross into a wooded trail. The young'uns stopped and drank of the water while Mom stood guard. Then these masked nightriders filed up to the ridge into the woods, disappearing into the sunrise.

Being awake to life's gifts has taken considerable relearning on my part. It was easier to be *busy* and put on my blinders always having to get the next job done. Talk about taking the joy out of the journey. My mother had told me over and over, "You learned to run before you walked." She said, "Slow down."

But I'd been a stubborn child and a stubborn adult refusing to walk to anyone's slowing beat. When I did read or play alone for hours, even those choices were all consuming. I gobbled books whole. I swam repetitive laps until I was a chlorinated prune. It drove my mother to distraction. "You'll wear yourself out." She'd shoo me outside to leisurely ride my bike for "my own good."

Mother would be pleased that I'd at last heeded her advice. I did go outside and ride now, every day. I was grateful to do so. She'd also be pleased that I was writing again, this daughter who badgered her for a desk.

My grandmother, who'd sat in her castle window, had wanted me to sew, create. I thought she'd probably like my view and photographs. I liked playing with color, composition, and lines. I thanked her for her example of living with light and as an artist.

My husband, Andy, had said early in our courtship that he admired my mind. "I don't think I'd ever be bored living with you." I think I must have become very boring when I became a work-a-holic and crashed in the recliner night after night. But I'm not so boring anymore. Andy's words helped me keep my faith in us and in myself.

For my sixtieth birthday, Andy presented me with a new bike with good brakes and two saddlebags. I was excited as any six-year-old with a new set of wheels to ride. The saddlebags have been filled with camera, pens, and paper. The views from my studio, in my journal, from my friends, and from my bike seat would nourish me pulling me out of life's tight places when I was a cantankerous, old bear. I'd continue to ride, play, and sing my hosannas. The Emerald Necklace beckoned.

Appendix: Carole's Diabetic Prediction Path (CDPP)

Behavior/ Feeling Challenge: Not Writing, Out of Touch with Inner Cravings

Trigger	Intervention	Do Now	Life-Long
1. No regular writing routine.	1. Schedule one hour daily.	1. Find Pen & Paper.	1. Journal every day.
2. Get too busy. "No time" refrains	2. First hour of the morning	2. No excuses. Get busy writing.	2. Remember what's important.
3. Get distracted and do laundry. Do anything, but write.	3. Emulate Natalie Goldberg & leave house.	3. Cafes waiting. Find one. Use library.	3. Laundry can wait. Writing can't.
4. Feel drained.	4. Do warm-up prompts. Don't give in.	4. Read Ueland & other writers on writing.	4. Surround self with other writers.
5. Not good enough. No talent.	5. Practice makes better. Think of self not as a leisure but a serious writer. Intention and persistence are everything.	5. Go to writing workshops. Read good writing. Learn.	5. Don't let the process toss me away. Believe in gift that is inside.

Behavior / Feeling Challenge: Eating Seconds

Trigger	Intervention	Do Now	Life-Long
1. When tastes good.	1. Slow down, Savor first serving.	1. Put away leftovers before sit down to eat.	1. Shrink stomach.
2. When still hungry.	2. Have a bottle of Water. Get up & go for a walk. Read for awhile. Have clear soup.	2. Tell self can have the second helping at the next meal. If still hungry, have some celery.	2. Remember my brain doesn't feel full, until a **full** hour after eating

Trigger	Intervention	Do Now	Life Long
3. Rebellion.	3. Learn difference between habit & hunger. Drink a glass of iced water. Chew ice cubes. Crush water, not self.	3. Only make a single serving meal. Get out ten raisins & chew slowly.	3. Eat Mind-Fully. Reactivate the volatiles.

Behavior / Feeling Challenge: *What's The Use* **Blues?**
Non-Edible Blood Sugar Highs

Trigger	Intervention	Do Now	Life Long
Sickness & Stress	1. Stay with food plan, lessen intake.	1. Sleep/rest.	1. Be humble. Pray.
	2. Stay away from fruit juices. Drink herbal teas, diet drinks, water.	2. Sip water & read children's books.	2. Remember sickness & stress are a part of living.
	3. Eating is not a cure. Makes me feel blotto.	3. Know conditions not improved by eating cake, drinking milk shakes.	3. Remember *The Velveteen Rabbit.* Find your legs through loving actions.
	4. Check blood levels often. Consult doctor if get into trouble.	4. Write outrageous letters, but don't drop them in the mailbox.	4. Whisper promises about what will do when well again.
	5. Meditate. Sew. Collage. Handwork is Settling.	5. Take mental health day. Play.	5. Read memoirs on how others handle sickness, stressful episodes

Behavior/Feeling Challenge: Sabotaging Self & Progress with Old Excuses

When Occurs	Intervention	Do Right Now	Life-Long Behavior
1. Good lab results or weight loss leading to smug slippage.	1. Stay awake Recognize old patterns of behavior. Learn from mistakes.	1. Keep taking regular blood sugar readings. Don't beat self up. Get back to wellness behaviors pronto.	1. Persistence is key to success. Being successful is paved with sound habits. Showing up counts as 80%.
2. Listening & believing when someone says, "One bite won't hurt."	2. Tell saboteurs. the magic words, "I'm Diabetic."	2. Look in the mirror. Rejoice in changes. Strut. Remember *Saturday Night Live.*	2. Listen to your inner voice &. act well.
3. Too tired to exercise. Want to lounge..... vegetate.	3. Bike in a.m. Every day. If miss a morning workout, use exercise tapeor walk in the evening.	3. Do it faithfully. No excuses. Get moving. "Now is the hour..."	. Daily workout keeps the body strong and the mind relaxed.

Behavior / Feeling Challenge: Fast Food Orders

Trigger	Intervention	Do Now	Life-Long
1. During the work week.	1. Restaurant sit-down lunch of broiled fish & veggies.	1. Shop for fresh fruits & vegetables. Stock freezer with single serving meals.	1. Prepare ahead & take new choices to work.
2. No time to "fix" proper meal "mentality."	2. Keep cereal in bottom desk drawer. Have someone pick up a milk.	2. Order salad, chili, or yogurt at drive thru's. Go home & chill out.	2. Experiment. Observe skinny people's eating habits. Imitate them.

3. Craving for French fries, hamburgers.	3. Have one or the other, but not both.	3. Find a deli and find satisfying, healthy substitutes.	3. A healthy lunch, improves thinking abilities. Productive afternoons. Catnaps not needed.
4. Grown-ups get to eat out.	4. Pack a lunch to have readily available.	4. Re-think what grown-ups do.	4. Make time for a good lunch.

Behavior / Feeling Challenge: Eating Popcorn for Comfort

Trigger	Intervention	Do Now	Life-Long
1. If have my way, daily.	1. Abstinence.	1. Get popcorn out of the house.	1. Popcorn is not a need, it is a want!
2. Use to fill up. Satiate self.	2. Fill self up with something Else.	2. Chew on celery, gum.	2. Popcorn produces blood sugar Highs.
3. Automatic association with movies.	3. Enjoy movie for itself.	3. No movie if popcorn present.	3. Let go. Practice Abstinence.
4. Snack time.	4. Relax by rubbing hands and legs with fragrant lotion. Find a rocking chair.	4. If present, throw it to to the birds!	4. Ban it for life! Substitute other comfort foods/actions. Pet the cat.

Behavior / Feeling Challenge: New Image Fears & Confusions

Trigger	Intervention	Do Now	Life-Long
1.Each ten pound weight loss.	1. Don't get scared or smug	1.Buy new outfit. Weed out closet.	1. Bask in praise & good reflections.
2. Blood sugar normalized. A1c count a six.	2. Stay alert & assertive.	2. Trip to beauty spa, woods, or zoo; & not bakery.	2. *Thank you* rejoicing.
3. Loss of matron, keeper of the keys, in charge image.	3. Find support needed. Don't listen to detractors: *"Are you sick?"* *"Is something wrong?"*	3. Take photos & journal *snapshots of successes.*	3. Remember exercised muscles are more solid than lots of weight.
	4. Validate new self. Stand tall.	4. Enjoy health, improved energy.	4. To change is to be Alive!
	5. If too scared wear some oversized clothing & hide-out for awhile.	5. Practice affirmations: *I am strong & flexible.*	5. Imagine how good life can be looking like a Showgirl for special occasions.

Some Suggested Readings

Buscaglia, Leo. *The Fall of Freddie the Leaf.* Thorofare, New Jersey: Slack Incorporated, Distributed by Henry Holt and Company, 1982. This book is dedicated to all children who have ever suffered a permanent loss, and to the grownups who could not find a way to explain it.

Baker, Russell, *The Good Times.* New York: William Morrow and Company, Inc., 1989. Russell writes a memoir as his mother's ghost continues to haunt him. *It there's one thing I can't stand, it's a quitter."* Russell shares his pitfalls and triumphs as a journalist.

Cameron, Julia. *The Artist's Way.* New York, NY: A Jeremy P. Tarcher/Putnam Book, 1992. A book on reclaiming personal creativity complete with imaginative exercises.

Clark, Jean Illsley. *Self-Esteem: A Family Affair.* Minneapolis: Winston Press, 1978. This book is a classic about self-esteem and how to nurture it between children and grown-ups. The author believes that self-esteem is possibly the most essential ingredient for human happiness.

Dominguez, Joe and Vicki Robin. *Your Money or Your Life.* New York, NY: Penguin Books, 1993. Transforming a personal relationship with money and achieving financial independence.

Goldberg, Natalie. *Living Color.* New York, Toronto, London, Sydney, Auckland: Bantam Books, 1997. A writer paints her world and teaches us all about it's okay to take space for one's art.

Goldberg, Natalie. *Wild Mind.* New York, NY: A Bantam Book, November, 1990. This is the author's second book on living the writer's life.

Jung, C.G., *Memories, Dreams, Reflections,* edited by Aniela Faffe, New York: Vintage Books, 1965. Jung's thoughts on confrontations with the unconscious take on new meaning every time I read them. He also discusses that with increasing age, contemplation, and reflection, the inner images naturally play an ever greater part in man's life. "Your old men shall dream dreams."

Linnea, Ann. *Deep Water Passage—Spiritual Journey at Midlife*, New York: Pocketbook, 1997. Celebrating her 43rd birthday, Ann Linnea kayaked around Lake Superior in a 65-day journey of spiritual insight and awakening.

Longfellow, Henry Wadsworth, *Hiawatha.* New York, NY: Dial Books for Young Readers, 1983 edition. The epic poem written by Longfellow as *The Song of Hiawatha* is beautifully illustrated by Sandy Jeffers.

Milne, A.A. *Pooh Gets into a Tight Place,* New York, NY: E.P. Dutton & Co., Inc, 1926. A classic children's story for the greedy child within us all.

Moore, Thomas. *Meditations ... On the Monk Who Dwells in Daily Life,* New York: HarperCollins *Publishers,* 1994. A series of meditations to touch the spiritual monk who resides inside. Early monks went out to live in the desert to find emptiness. I needed to learn from the experts at how to do nothing and to nurture the culture of emptiness. I had the culture of *busyness* down pat and it was leaching me dry.

Murdock, Maureen. *The Heroine's Journey.* Boston & London: Shambhala, 1990. This book offers a map of the feminine healing process drawn from the author's experiences as a mother, artist, and therapist.

Pipher, Muriel. *Reviving Ophelia: Saving the Selves of Adolescent Girls,* New York: Ballantine, 1994. A psychologist and anthropologist, Dr. Pipher recommends creating a culture that has a place for every human gift. Using case studies, Pipher cautions adolescent girls against diminishing their sense of self.

Reichl, Ruth, *Tender At The Bone: Growing Up at the Table*, New York: Broadway Books, 1999. This well-crafted memoir is a classic for anyone who obsesses about food. Reichl discovered at an early age that "If you watched people as they ate, you could find out who they were." Her mother, the Queen of Mold, forces Reichl to learn how to cook, bake, and develop a delicious sense of humor.

Roth, Geneen. *Feeding The Hungry Heart.* New York, N.Y.: The Bobbs-Merrill Co., Inc., 1982. An inspirational book on healing the pain and isolation of compulsive eating.

See, Carolyn, *Making A Literary Life ... Advice for Writers and Other Dreamers.* New York: Random House, 2002. This writing guide not only teaches one how to write, it teaches how to live and survive the writing life.

Sendak, Maurice, *Where The Wild Things Are*, New York: Harper & Row Publishers, 1963. "And now," cried Max, "let the wild rumpus start!" This classic children's book on being out-of-control is blessing for the angry me. And after the temper tantrum was over, Max was still in his room and his supper was still hot. This book always gives hope.

Shulman, Alix Kates. *Drinking The Rain.* New York, NY: Farrar, Straus and Giroux, 1995. Building a new life of creativity and spirituality, self-reliance and self-fulfillment at fifty.

Williams, Margary. *The Velveteen Rabbit.* New York: Doubleday & Company, Inc., 1922. This classic children's tale tells the story of how to become *real* through love.

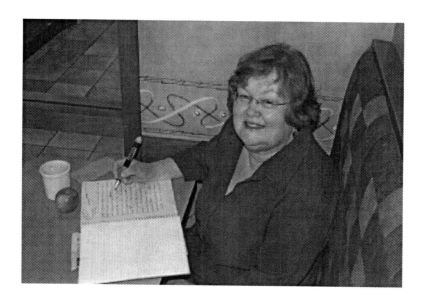

Carole Calladine, MSSA, LISW, is a clinical social worker with over thirty years of experience. Now in the second half of life, she writes out of an innate fascination about relationships, life stages, and choices. She is a gifted family life educator in print and in person. Her masters degree in social service administration is from Case Western Reserve University and her undergraduate honors degree in sociology is from the State University of Iowa.

Second Story Woman is her third book, following *Raising Siblings ...Raising Brothers and Sisters Without Raising the Roof,* on sibling rivalry, and *One Terrific Year...Supporting Your Kids Through the Ups and Downs of Their Year,* on the repetitive themes of childhood. For seven years, she wrote *You and Your Teen-Ager* for the Sunday edition of *The Cleveland Plain Dealer.* The author is an educator and keynote speaker at conferences from New York to British Columbia. She specializes in facilitating workshops on wellness, creativity, and writing.

An avid bicycler, the author resides with her husband, Andrew, in a house overlooking the Cleveland Metroparks and its biking trails. Currently, she is the Director of Senior Services for the City of Rocky River where seniors enjoy opportunities for second stories.

Bird Dog Publishing

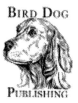

Second Story Woman: A Memoir of Second Chances
by Carole Calladine
978-1-933964-12-6   226 pgs. $15.00

Another Life: Collected Poems by Allen Frost
978-1-933964-10-2   176 pgs. $14.00

Winter Apples: Poems by Paul S. Piper
978-1-933964-08-9   88 pgs. $14.00

Lake Effect: Poems by Laura Treacy Bentley
1-933964-05-7   108 pgs. $14.00

Faces and Voices: Tales by Larry Smith
1-933964-04-9   136 pgs. $14.00

Depression Days on an Appalachian Farm: Poems
by Robert L. Tener
1-933964-03-0   80 pgs. $14.00

120 Charles Street, The Village:
Journals & Other Writings 1949-1950 by Holly Beye
0-933087-99-3   240 pgs. $15.00

Bird Dog Publishing
PO 425/ Huron, OH 44839
http://members.aol.com/Lsmithdog/bottomdog/BirdDogPage.html
A division of Bottom Dog Press, Inc.

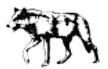

CPSIA information can be obtained at www.ICGtesting.com
Printed in the USA
BVOW03s1838020415

394525BV00002B/127/P